A Tiger by the Tail

A Tiger by the Tail

Berthajane Vandegrift

Writers Club Press
San Jose New York Lincoln Shanghai

A Tiger by the Tail

Writers Club Press
an imprint of iUniverse, Inc.

For information address:
iUniverse, Inc.
5220 S. 16th St., Suite 200
Lincoln, NE 68512
www.iuniverse.com

ISBN: 0-595-20471-6

Printed in the United States of America

Dedication

To my children, grandchildren and great grandchildren. While none of the latter have yet been conceived, I would value such an intimate account by one of my ancestors.

CONTENTS

INTRODUCTION

Psychiatrists once believed that virtually all mental illness was caused by bad parenting. This included schizophrenia, alcoholism, and even homosexuality. Bruno Bettelheim, a well-known psychologist, declared "maternal rejection" to be the cause of developmental disabilities such as autism and Asperger's Syndrome.

A Tiger by the Tail is a personal account of a "disturbed" child, and the therapy to which our family was subjected.

Mothers of autistic children are no longer accused of maternal rejection, and medical science no longer subjects people to psychotherapy as a treatment for mental illness. However much of the public still accepts the Freudian notion that subconscious feelings and emotions can damage "psyches".

Psychologists claiming to have some mysterious special understanding of human motivation that the rest of us lack promote such syndromes as "repressed memory", "multiple personality", and "Munchhausen by Proxy". As long as people are viewed as consisting of materialistic entities such as "psyches", "ids", "egos" and "superegos", and the public believes complex human behavior can be reduced to such materialistic formulas, we will remain vulnerable to a psychology industry competing for a shrinking market.

CHAPTER I

A Strange Checkup

"Tell me about yourself," the young pediatrician said. Wearing a starched white coat over his Army uniform, he sat behind his desk regarding me gravely through horn-rimmed glasses. I stared back, baffled. It sounded like something a psychiatrist might say. But this doctor was a pediatrician, not a psychiatrist! The silence became uncomfortable. The partitions of the Army clinic were flimsy, and I could hear a buzz of activity out in the crowded waiting room.

I always dreaded talking to doctors. Army clinics were busy, and in those days we didn't consult a doctor for colds and minor problems. Doctors seemed intimidating authority figures with mysterious powers to cure obscure, life-threatening illnesses. I often felt obligated to convince a doctor my particular illness was serious. However on this particular occasion no one was sick, and I hadn't arrived at the pediatrician's office in my usual state of anxiety. I'd brought my three-year-old son to the clinic, not because I thought something was wrong with him, but because a neighbor had suggested it. I would have felt foolish admitting I'd brought my child to a doctor simply because of a neighbor, so I explained Tony didn't talk much, was still in diapers, and maybe he should have a checkup. Instead of examining Tony, the doctor kept trying to initiate personal conversation.

"How do you like the new administration in Washington?" he asked. "It's exciting, isn't it?"

"Society will be in trouble unless people start taking responsibility for their own lives," the doctor said. "People expect the government to do everything for them."

I admired Kennedy, our young new president, but apparently this doctor and I would disagree on politics. I sat silently waiting for him to begin examining Tony.

"Tell me about yourself," he said again.

Tony was busy examining the contents of the wastebasket. "Sometimes Tony's temper can get pretty violent," I finally said, hoping to return the doctor's attention to his patient. Maybe one of Tony's glands needed adjusting or something.

"Does he understand what you say to him?" the doctor asked.

"I'm never sure. He rarely does what I tell him, but he's independent and stubborn."

Tony was on his knees, his little blue-jean-clad rear end up in the air and his head on the floor, trying to see under a partition into the next office. If anyone were on the other side of that partition, they'd probably feel uncomfortable to see his bright, inquisitive little face peeking up at them. I picked him up and held him on my lap.

"How does he get along with other children?"

"I don't think I've noticed him play with other children."

"Does he have opportunities to be around them?"

"Off and on, I guess. Come to think of it, he doesn't play with his brother and sister very much."

"Where do you live?"

"In a big old house on a hill behind San Rafael."

"You own your home?" I nodded.

"You are lucky to own property in such a valuable area."

He seemed to expect a response, so I tried to think of one.

"The house is a hundred years old and has termites," I said. "In the coming depression, it probably won't be worth what we paid for it."

"We don't have depressions any more," the doctor scoffed.

Many of us who grew up during the thirties, sometimes accused of having depression mentalities, didn't really trust prosperity, but the doctor's comment seemed condescending.

"You are probably too young to know what a depression is," I said. The doctor frowned. I was startled by my own impertinence. Suffering from shyness, I was rarely rude or impudent. Perhaps the doctor was making an effort to be friendly. Army doctors were not known for a bedside manner, but I'd never before encountered one with either time or inclination for such personal conversation.

"Tell me about your husband," he said after a moment. Tony slid off my lap to examine the scales. Again, I was baffled. I couldn't imagine why our personal lives might be of concern to this pediatrician. Surely he wasn't interested in Ike's vital statistics, such as height, weight or eye-color.

"He's stationed in Greenland right now," I said.

"Uh-oh! That's bad."

That was a strange comment for an Army doctor to make. There was nothing unusual about overseas duty in military families. I eyed the doctor silently, and he continued.

"How do you feel about your husband's absence?"

"Well he'll be home in a couple of months."

The doctor glanced at Tony. After trying to turn the valves under the sink, Tony had crawled onto a bookcase. With a self-satisfied smile, he crouched n the bottom shelf like a life-sized cherubic bookend.

"Ever since you came, your little boy has been running around the office examining the equipment. He's paid no attention to me. Why, he's hardly aware I'm in the room!"

You haven't done anything but talk, I thought, and Tony doesn't understand much of that. However I wasn't accustomed to arguing with doctors, and I nodded.

"Your child is not normal," he said.

"You really think so?"

His words seemed to have no impact. After all, he hadn't examined Tony I listened to the doctor make another appointment for us, but I was puzzling over what on earth this peculiar pediatrician had been up to for the past half-hour.

The age of scientific materialism may have begun with Descartes, but in 1961, with the atomic bomb a fearsome recent event, materialism had taken possession of popular thinking. The universe was believed to be composed of bits of matter, interacting with each other according to measurable, impersonal "laws". The simplistic, mechanical formula, "random mutation and natural selection", was believed to have accidentally created a purposeless diversity of nature, and similar mechanistic laws were being sought to explain and measure the mind. Psychiatry was confident that with Freudian analysis, it had found the psychological equivalent of E equals M,C squared. However, while most of America was obsessed with psychiatry, it was not one of my interests. I had heard of Freud. (I wasn't yet aware of many of Freud's discoveries, such as his assertion that masturbation, condoms and suppressed sexual fantasies cause impotence, consumption, paralysis, seizures and insanity.) I was vaguely aware that psychiatrists were trained medical experts devising scientific methods for repairing malfunctioning psyches. While I was uncertain of the definition of a "psyche", I assumed there was nothing wrong with mine.

My ignorance of psychiatry would soon be remedied. Autism, of which I'd never heard, was considered to be the result of "maternal rejection". Treatment consisted of therapists (usually men) conducting an investigation to determine why mother was rejecting her child—but trying to speak in terms that disguised the offensive nature of their accusation. I had no premonition of what was about to happen to us as I left the doctor's office that day. I was an ordinary housewife and mother, easily intimidated by everyone but small children and other housewives. I was forty years old, and the second half of my life was about to begin. Our up-coming therapy would change me, all right, but not in ways the therapists were hoping. While resisting the psychologists' attempts to convince me something was wrong with my psyche, I would develop a confidence of which I never dreamed I was capable.

CHAPTER 2

Who is more devastated, the disabled child or the parent?

Pondering the pediatrician's strange behavior, I drove home. Like many mothers bringing their children to the Army clinic, I had dressed casually—in slacks. People had told me I had a nice smile, but I didn't smile much around doctors, and I doubted there was anything unusual about my appearance to evoke the pediatrician's curiosity. I'd simply taken my little boy for a checkup. But instead of examining Tony, the doctor acted as if I were the patient—as though he suspected something might be wrong with me. He even seemed to have questions about Tony's father, who was way up in Greenland.

A light spring rain was falling when we arrived home to our big, old three-story, shingled house. On our way up the brick walk, some drops of water fell from the redwood trees and hit Tony on the face. He looked up at the dripping leaves and laughed, his big blue eyes sparkling with delight. His laughter was happy and infectious, and I laughed too. At nearly four, Tony was the healthiest, and most handsome of our three children. He even looked boyishly adorable wearing his stained, faded old sweater. This scruffy looking garment had to be draped over him carefully. In spite of constant mending there always seemed to be holes other than the sleeves through which he could put his arms. He didn't wear his sweater for warmth; he was comfortable outside on the coldest days in nothing but a diaper. However Tony was a determined child, and he refused to go anywhere without this cherished, shabby looking bunch of yarn. He was also a mischievous little rascal with an active imagination and uncontrollable curiosity. One day as we walked along a street, Tony suddenly squatted down and peeked up under a lady's skirt. She squealed in alarm and jumped back.

"Tony!" I exclaimed.

The woman noticed Tony's puzzled expression and seemed to regain some of her composure.

"I suppose he thought one good peek was better than guessing," she conceded.

A few days later I noticed Tony start toward two nuns in long black habits. Fearing nuns might not be as casual about Tony's peeking, I ran and caught him by the hand. The nuns smiled indulgently, unaware of what Tony may have had in mind.

At times Tony's curiosity could lure him into frightening situations. One morning I awoke to see him walking along the narrow roof over-hang outside our third-floor, bedroom window. Creeping up to the window, fearful of startling him, I reached carefully out and snatched him back into the safety of the room. Tony laughed, for he loved to roughhouse. We quickly nailed heavy screens over the windows, but he discovered other ways onto the roof, such as climbing from the balustrade of an upstairs porch. However Tony never harmed himself by any of his dangerous stunts.

My older children arrived home from school soon after Tony and I returned from the doctor. Guy was in the third grade. A quiet, reflective little boy by nature, he had recently begun to express a dislike for school. His answer to my question, "What happened in school today?" was the usual "Nothin'".

Sherry, my little six-year-old, was breathlessly bubbling with excitement. "I told Guy ghost stories on the way home," she said.

"Did you frighten him?"

"No, but I sure scared myself."

My mind still on the pediatrician, I smiled absently.

The children ate bananas for after-school snacks. Tony's broke, and he erupted into violent, angry sobs. He furiously tried to stick the two pieces back together, mashing them to a gooey pulp. His temper was like a small tornado. It could subside in an instant, and he'd be all smiles and sparkling blue eyes again. Some trivial annoyance might cause such a storm.

For instance, one evening we were eating corn on the cob. Maybe some of it stuck between Tony's teeth. In any case, he suddenly hurled the corn across the room, followed by his plate of food, and his glass of milk flew over our heads and spattered against the wall. By the time we had recovered from our shock and captured him, Tony was furiously slinging food in all directions. A few minutes later, while we were still wiping up the mashed potatoes, Tony laughed, his rage having evaporated.

Guy and Sherry never had temper tantrums, and I hadn't yet figured out how to handle Tony's. I took the banana he was angrily trying to repair and gave him another. He consumed it contentedly, tears of fury still glimmering on his beautiful long lashes.

All afternoon I remained preoccupied over my strange visit to the pediatrician. When I called the children to dinner that evening, Tony came in from the yard walking backwards. He backed through the house and up to the table. He tried to sit in his highchair backwards, but found that unpractical, and turned around to await his dinner. The week before, Tony had draped a towel over his head so he couldn't see, and spent the day groping his way around the house and yard. Those were the types of games he played.

He also spent hours creating beautiful, intricate designs with a set of multi-shaped, colored blocks. He seemed indifferent to our admiration of his creations, but apparently got some personal satisfaction from building them. He was always busy, and when we came across a banana skin, a pencil and a toothpaste cap laid out on the floor in the shape of an airplane, we'd smile and recognize Tony had been at work.

It was this artistic inclination that finally got him into trouble. Tony redesigned a neighbor's garden. He pulled up all the flowers she had planted the day before and rearranged them, with their roots exposed, in a new symmetrical pattern. I sympathized with my neighbor's outrage, and paddled Tony when I caught him in her yard. Spanking only seemed to make Tony angry, and he'd furiously haul off and kick a tree or rock. He'd even come and bend over for his spanking when I caught him next door, but punishment did not keep him home. He appeared to become more determined. After watching my futile efforts for a couple of days, my neighbor's anger subsided somewhat.

"Have you taken him to a doctor?" she asked.

"What on earth could a doctor do about it?"

She stood watching Tony without answering.

There was no medical cure for mischievousness, independence and determination, and those would be silly reasons to take a kid to a doctor. Besides, I wasn't worried because Tony was slow to talk and toilet-train. My older son had been slow to mature and was now a delightful little nine-year old. Nevertheless, friends had appeared shocked by some of Tony's antics. Maybe everyone would be more tolerant of him if I could tell them the medical profession had pronounced him normal. I called a nearby military hospital and made an appointment. Five hours had passed now since that appointment.

An uneasy, murky fear was beginning to gnaw at me as I stood at the kitchen sink washing the dinner dishes.

Tony had a number of fears. We became aware of his reaction to loud noises when we rented a floor sander. Tony didn't cry when we turned it on; he butted the screen door open with his head and left home. He was barely a year old and couldn't walk, but was speeding down the walk on his hands and knees when we caught up with him.

Tony was terrified of barbers. He was a masculine appearing child, and no one would have mistaken him for a girl. Nevertheless, long hair would have been unacceptable on a boy before the 1960's, so I bought clippers and tried to cut his hair myself. I would sneak up on him but never managed to do more than a partial job before he escaped, leaving him with a ragged, ever-changing hair style.

New clothes, especially new shoes, frightened him. Recently I had bought him a pair in a department store. His loud protests embarrassed me, but even in his tattered old sweater, Tony looked cute and evoked sympathy.

"Poor little boy," commented other customers.

"What's wrong with the little fellow?"

"Don't you like those pretty new shoes, dear?" asked a saleslady, kneeling in front of him.

Tony shoved her away and kicked over a display rack, scattering shoes all over the floor. I apologized, and then followed as he marched indignantly from the store, wailing with rage and still clutching his dirty old shoes in his little fists. The new shoes disappeared that night. My neighbor found them a few days later, hidden in her hedge.

Guy had many of the same fears and outgrew them, I reminded myself, and loud noises had always frightened me.

Suddenly that obscure uneasiness hidden in the recesses of my mind exploded into consciousness.

The doctor said my child was not normal!

Regardless of how strangely the doctor had behaved, he was a pediatrician. We all wanted to believe doctors knew everything—could fix anything. Such an authority would surely never declare a child was abnormal without being certain.

It might seem strange that I had no immediate reaction to the doctor's declaration, but I have since come to realize my emotional reactions are often delayed. If someone insults me, for instance, I don't feel offended until later. When in shock my mind seems to work in slow motion. Although I was forty years old, this was the most shocking news I'd ever had to confront. For five hours I'd ignored it. The children were in bed, and I was alone. Ike was in Greenland, and I'd never felt so alone. I began to cry.

Vaguely aware children might have *emotional problems*, I didn't know what the term meant. *Emotional problems* must surely have some connection with unhappiness. I remembered Tony's delightful laughter. He was obviously a happy child, and his trouble couldn't be emotional. The pediatrician must have meant Tony was mentally retarded.

I cried through that long, lonely night.

Why was I grieving like this? It couldn't be for Tony. Unaware anything had happened he was in bed sleeping as peacefully as the night before. The doctor's declaration that Tony wasn't normal hadn't changed my little boy. At dinner he had been my same delightful, self-confident Tony. All this anguish surely couldn't be for myself. How could self-pity cause this much pain?

Maybe I was grieving for some little boy who had never existed—except in my imagination. That little boy would have lived whatever wonderful life he chose. He would have had the ability to face life's challenges of life, and grow up to—

—to do what? What *did* I wish for my children?

Maybe I had some vague hope Sherry would find a nice man to take care of her and provide her with material possessions, such as cars and swimming pools. Yet that wasn't what I had sought for myself. Perhaps I had secret visions of my sons becoming rich and famous. Yet fame and fortune hadn't been my priority in life. Most parents claim they simply want their children to be happy. But what did that mean? Could anyone even recognize happiness without having experienced unhappiness? In any case, retardation wouldn't necessarily cause Tony to be unhappy.

So why was I crying like this?

After forty years of pondering the question, I now know what I wish for my children. (and grandchildren). I hope they develop the strength, and become tough enough to deal with all the problems, frustrations, tragedies and disappointments that are a part of all normal "happy" lives. However, as I struggled to face the possibility that Tony might not lead a normal life, I continued to cry. Since the imaginary Tony was apparently gone, I tried to think of my Tony, the little boy in bed asleep, as a retarded adult. Surely I would love him too.

I remembered a retarded man my husband's grandmother had raised. Rutledge was his name, and he was usually cheerful. He was a competent farmhand and played the harmonica at local barn dances. When I knew Rutledge, Ike's grandmother was past eighty and alone except for him. She and Rutledge needed each other. With his limited understanding, Rutledge often seemed to find the world more interesting and exciting than many people with greater ability did. When he was well past sixty, we heard him say to Ike's grandmother,

"Gee, Mama, it's going to be a lucky girl who gets me for a husband, isn't it, Mama? I don't drink or stay out late or waste my money, like Jim and those other boys do. Isn't that right, Mama? Isn't it going to be a lucky girl that gets me, Mama?" We all laughed with him. How could anyone feel sorry for such an enthusiastic sixty-year-old?

I was unable to think of Tony growing up to be retarded. I'd always had the feeling Tony might be like Ike's grandfather, a doctor, who seemed to have made a profound impression upon people. His patients regarded him with an awe that lasted long after his death. Ike's father wrote a book about him, and everyone who had known him talked about him and quoted him. The many anecdotes about Ike's grandfather, whom I'd never met, made him seem a revered, legendary figure of Ike's family. Tony resembled a baby picture I had of this esteemed doctor, but I wondered now if I'd believed Tony was like him from an unconscious realization that Tony himself was different—and mysterious.

Dawn brought an end to that long sleepless night. I looked out the window at the redwoods and bay trees growing on our ivy-covered hillside. Our yard and the neighbor's garden, which Tony had redesigned, looked the same in the cold, misty, morning light. I shivered. My life seemed changed forever during that dark, bleak night alone in a rumpled bed. Yesterday morning I'd jumped out of it, ready for the day ahead. Would I ever again face life with the same eager attitude?

CHAPTER 3

Is all that science cannot measure fictitious?

I kept trying to think of Tony as mentally retarded. Retarded people lived in institutions. If Tony were in such a place, maybe I could forget him. My little boy would no longer be a part of my life, but I might eventually escape from this relentless grief. The thought of abandoning Tony to a state hospital couldn't possibly have increased the anguish I was already suffering. That morning after Sherry and Guy left for school, I called the pediatric clinic.

"I spoke with a doctor there yesterday, a pediatrician. I don't remember his name," I said to the woman who answered. "Maybe he had blond hair and wore glasses."

"What did you talk to him about?"

"My little boy. The doctor said—well—I guess he said Tony was mentally retarded." I began to cry again. "Somehow, I didn't realize what the doctor meant yesterday."

"Try not to worry," she said. "Give me your name. I'll find out which doctor and have him call you."

I put down the phone and looked out the window at Tony playing in the yard.

Oh Tony, please do something clever! These past few hours must surely be a nightmare from which I will awaken. Tragedies like this happened to other people, not us. I can't explain why I thought we should be exempt.

Tony came in and emptied two pockets of dirt out of his little trousers onto the floor.

"Oh, Tony," I scolded.

Tony picked up the edge of the rug, kicked the dirt under it, and looked up at me inquiringly. Ever since rugs were invented people have thought it clever to sweep dirt under them, but Tony's ingenuity dispelled none of my despair, and I hugged him to me unhappily.

After a while the pediatrician called.

"When you said yesterday Tony wasn't normal, the meaning didn't seem to register. I'm sorry."

"But I didn't say he was mentally retarded," the doctor objected.

"You didn't?"

"No. Actually, I suspect his trouble might be something quite different."

"If you mean some emotional problem, I wish I could believe that. It's not true of Tony. He's a happy child."

"Don't feel too discouraged yet," he said. "Come in again next week. We'll try to get your little boy an appointment at a psychiatric clinic."

A psychiatric clinic? Where psychiatrists do whatever they do? I vaguely imagined those mysterious medical specialists sitting silently, listening to a patient on a couch describing his dreams. From a few obscure clues, they could scientifically detect people's deepest subconscious thoughts. They also had formulae to measure a child's intelligence more accurately than any fallible human judgment could. Although a few things existed that science hadn't yet learned to measure, those of us who believed in science knew anything "real" was measurable. Human traits, such as intelligence, were obviously neither fictitious nor imaginary, and surely by this time psychiatrists had devised scientific methods to measure them. Psychiatrists also delved into a person's past, didn't they? Tony didn't have much of a past, but I thought over the few years of his life.

*   *   *

Ike was a major in the Army, and we had two children. I enjoyed the life of an Army wife. We moved every couple of years, and each new post was different. After a European tour of duty, we were stationed in Colorado. The fishing was wonderful, but after hectic days of pulling toddlers out of streams and rescuing them from falling down banks, I left the fishing to Ike. We bought a small house, our first, and I tended a yard full of flowers. Planning to have two children, a boy and then a girl, I felt disgusted to find myself pregnant at the age of thirty-seven. If abortions had been legal, I would have had one. Nevertheless, something (I've since read it was hormones) soon convinced me a baby was a good idea. By my fourth month, I was eagerly looking forward to another child. Guy and Sherry came down with measles. I was sure I'd had them as a child, but the doctor gave me a shot of gamma globulin, which was supposed to lighten the illness in case I hadn't. There was nothing unusual about Tony's delivery. *Bastille Day* was probably an appropriate date to launch us upon those next turbulent decades, for Tony was born on July 14, 1957. He arrived several weeks early, on a Sunday, and Ike had gone fishing. Leaving the children with a neighbor, I took a taxi to the hospital, where I discovered my doctor had also gone fishing. The baby didn't wait for my doctor. Tony was born after a few hours, and my first question was the same one most mothers ask,

"Is the baby all right?"

"A fine healthy boy," the substitute doctor said from behind a surgical mask. Such was my faith in medical science, I assumed the doctor had determined Tony's normalcy in that first glance. I never gave the matter another thought.

When Tony was sixteen months old, Ike was sent to an artillery school in Oklahoma for a few months. He had orders for Korea after he finished the school. The children and I went to California to stay near my family.

I'd suspected a two-day train trip in a cramped little compartment with three small children might not be fun. It wasn't. The two older ones bickered to relieve their boredom. Tony, the only one who seemed to enjoy himself, jumped up and down on my lap. He made a mess every meal, even breaking a bottle of catsup and spilling it over us all. I stole moments of relief by ordering a cup of coffee and locking myself in the tiny toilet. If the designers of railroad cars had anticipated mothers might use that little closet to escape rambunctious toddlers and bickering children, they would have surely made it larger.

In California, I rented a house next door to my sister. Her husband's work kept him away from home much of the time.

"My children resent their father being away", she said. "Yours will become unhappy too." Believing one of the obligations of parenthood was to avoid unhappiness, I thought of ways to keep us busy.

"I don't understand it," my sister said a few weeks later. "Your children are eager for their father to get home, but they don't seem unhappy." She probably meant I didn't appear unhappy. Her children seemed all right to me, and I suspected she was the one who resented her husband's absence.

My sister once took Tony to town to buy him a toy. Tony could not be talked into anything. He shook his head and responded a decisive "No!" to everything she offered. Awed by Tony's determination, she took him into a big toy store and told the clerks she would buy anything in which they could interest her nephew. She spent an entertaining afternoon as they exhibited their most expensive toys. Despite the clerks' enthusiastic demonstrations, Tony continued to shake his head and declare a determined "No!" My sister left the store without a purchase. We laughed when she told about it

Our yard was always full of children. As I remembered the doctor asking how Tony got along with other children, I realized Tony never paid much attention to them. If the other children played in the sandbox, Tony played on the swings, and vice versa. He would roam out of the yard. I would find him, scold him, and give him a swat on the diaper. Once, we couldn't find him anywhere. After frantically searching the neighborhood, we called the police. Someone several blocks away had found him, and two policemen brought Tony home frightened, tearful and sobbing,

"Tony broke! Tony broke!" *Broke* was one of the few words in his vocabulary.

Like my older son, Tony had not babbled as a baby. His first words were 'see boat'. No one knew the reason for his fascination with boats, but we all joined his game and yelled, "See boat!" when we spotted a car pulling one along the freeway. However, except for a couple of familiar words or phrases, Tony was a silent observer. Mine was a family who enjoyed differences in people, including children. My four-year-old nephew insisted he had a herd of colored goats that were invisible to the rest of us. "You are sitting right on top of my green goat!" he would declare, causing startled visitors to jump up in alarm from wherever they were sitting. At other times my nephew claimed he was a robot and had to be wound up every morning. We assumed whatever our children did was normal, and often funny, and that assumption included any differences we noticed in Tony.

Ike returned from the school in Oklahoma. In a month he would leave for Korea, and we plunged into a flurry of activities with the children, such as fishing, picnics and going to zoos and museums. However I could see Ike was troubled. For one thing, he had purchased a swagger stick. A few officers sometimes carried this ridiculous little item around, for no other purpose as far as I could see, than to prop up their egos. I couldn't imagine Ike needing one. He had always been a public information officer, and the school he had attended was an artillery school. It had included mathematics and difficult, technical information. Ike admitted the course had not gone well.

A couple of weeks before he was to leave for Korea, what Ike had secretly feared and dreaded, happened. The armed forces had been cutting back, and orders arrived relieving him from active duty as an officer in the Army Reserve. That feeling of failure was one of the most painful things Ike ever had to endure, and my heart ached for him. However, we had always led a more eventful, unconventional life than most people, and we turned our attention to dealing with our altered circumstances. With only five years until retirement, Ike could enlist as a sergeant to finish his twenty years. Then he would retire as a major. At least now he didn't have to go to Korea. Although Ike and I were busy trying to adjust to a different future, the children were too young to pay much attention, and the event didn't have much effect upon them. Tony, not yet two, wasn't unaware anything was happening.

Ike enlisted at the Presidio at San Francisco. We bought a big old triplex across the Golden Gate Bridge in Marin County, renting out a couple of apartments. I was happy to try to think of ways to help with the finances. We lived a quiet, uneventful life until Ike was sent to Greenland eight months earlier. Temporary separations were routine in the Army, and the children and I went on with our lives while awaiting Ike's return.

★   ★   ★

I went for my next appointment with the pediatrician, but this time I was frightened. What happened that day might have been partly due to the snobbery of Army rank, which extended to wives in those days.

Captain's wives outranked lieutenant's wives, and the general's wife could tell us all what to do. Fraternization between officers and enlisted personnel was forbidden. Doctors were officers, and I was an enlisted wife. Also, in my emotional turmoil I had shown up dressed somewhat like a migrant farm worker. I did take *Castor Oil and Quinine*, the book about Tony's great grandfather. I think I hoped it might give substance to my vague belief Tony was unusual because he would grow up to have some mysterious quality like Dr. Vandegrift. Tony was not precocious, but I'd decided precocious children didn't necessarily grow up to be the most capable adults, and apparently Dr. Vandegrift had agreed. In fact, Tony's great grandfather was quoted as recommending children not start school until the age of eight in order to guard against early intellectual development. Perhaps late bloomers ran in the family.

The pediatrician's hair was dark, not blond, I noticed. The words he had spoken were stark in my memory, but other details of the doctor's appearance had been blasted out of my mind.

He greeted me briefly, as though impatient to begin, with only a glance at Tony. He didn't mention the psychiatric appointment he had spoken of on the phone. Instead, he tenaciously continued with the same menacing demand of the previous week,

"Well now, tell me about yourself."

Weren't we going to even make a pretense of discussing Tony? I wanted to answer him, but somehow couldn't. I'd always found doctors intimidating, but I'd never encountered one so threateningly intrusive.

"If you have some wild idea you are going to get to know me, forget it! No one knows me as intimately as you seem to have in mind," I said. Then I sighed. "But for some reason I don't understand, this is supposedly for Tony. Go ahead. What do you want to know?"

"Just tell me anything you can think of."

The doctor apparently wanted me to rattle on about myself, saying whatever popped into my head. If I attempted such a thing I'd probably blurt out something inane. Was that what he hoped I would do?

In 1961 in the United States, the validity of this new science, psychiatry, was rarely challenged. Psychotherapy was prescribed as treatment for many ailments of unknown cause. Anyone who resisted such personal intrusion was contemptuously accused of refusing help. The doctor and I spent a half-hour verbally sparring, and I managed not to tell him much of anything. Tony, sensing my distress, stood and watched the doctor instead of pursuing his usual explorations, but like the previous week, the pediatrician ignored him. Finally, the despair on my face must have convinced the doctor I wasn't being intentionally difficult. He stopped and tried a fresh approach.

"Was your husband a sergeant when Tony was born?"

"No. He was a major. He was RIFF'ed a couple of years ago, but that did not cause us any terrible unhappiness. There are even advantages—such as not having to attend officers' wives' luncheons."

"You don't like officers' wives' luncheons?"

"No. Would you?"

He hesitated, and I detected a trace of smile at the corners of his mouth. Maybe I could distract him from badgering me for a minute.

"Well? How would you like to attend women's luncheons?"

His grin finally materialized. "I can't picture myself wearing the appropriate clothes," he said. He didn't stay distracted for long though, and soon resumed his relentless questioning.

"Everyone has their peculiarities," I said. Which of mine was this doctor so determined to expose? I would willingly confess to something if it would end this inquisition. "Maybe Tony is simply going to grow up to be peculiar like his great grandfather." I indicated the book I'd brought about Dr. Vandegrift.

"What was peculiar about him?"

I faltered. It would seem immodest to come right out and admit I thought my child was exceptionally intelligent, and I finally blurted out,

"Well, he was clairvoyant."

Tony's great grandfather was said to have once jumped up from the dinner table in New York and declared his barn in Maryland was on fire. It was. I was aware that extra sensory perception was not a respectable notion in our twentieth-century, scientific society, and like most modern, educated people, I didn't question science. I usually avoided thinking about Dr. Vandegrift's reported psychic abilities by deciding he was probably highly perceptive, and had somehow convinced everyone he was clairvoyant. To my relief the pediatrician ignored my suggestion and didn't ask me to explain. His seemed preoccupied with something else I'd said.

"Peculiar," he said. "Peculiar."

He stood up and walked over to the window. Then he turned and resumed questioning.

"Where did you grow up?"

"In Ukiah, a small town in Northern California."

"And your husband?"

"He's from New York."

"Where were you married?"

"We were married by a one-armed preacher in Alaska." I wasn't trying to be flippant. I merely thought this miserable ordeal might become less grim if we could inject a little levity into it.

"Alaska? What were you doing up there?"

"I don't know. Got restless, I guess."

"Restless," he said. "Restless…hmm. What type of work did you do in Alaska?"

"I've done lots of things. The first money I ever earned was selling acorns to Indians. In Alaska I made totem poles for the Indians."

"Totem poles! What did they do with them?"

"Burned them."

"Burned them?"

"Oh," I explained, exasperated at how seriously he took my attempts at humor, "I worked in a store. I carved some totem poles out of candles, and lots of people bought them, including some Indians."

He stood looming over me. It was probably just as well I hadn't told about getting into a poker game, down in the engine room, with the crew of the SS *North Sea*. When the ship reached Sitka, I didn't have enough money to come home if I had wanted.

"Architecture is what I studied in school," I said, sensing this was what he was trying to find out.

The doctor moved back toward his desk and was silent for a moment.

"Got pretty good grades, didn't you." It wasn't a question. He sounded less contentious, almost sympathetic.

"My grades were all right." They weren't quite as good as the doctor was making them sound.

"What is your religion. I mean—ah—do you have any religious affiliations?" A moment ago he had arrogantly badgered me to tell him details of my private life. Now, suddenly, he seemed embarrassed to ask my religion.

"Agnostic."

"Agnostic or atheist?"

"Agnostic I guess, but I send the children to Sunday school."

Most parents feel obligated to indoctrinate their children with their own theology. Resolving questions of one's personal philosophy, and finding meaning in twentieth century life, seemed to me the most difficult, significant accomplishment of anyone's life. Neither Ike nor I had any desire to impose our beliefs upon anyone else, including our children.

The doctor sat down at his desk and began writing in Tony's medical record.

"I'll try to get you an appointment at a psychiatric clinic as soon as possible, Mrs. Vandegrift," he said without looking up from the folder.

He appeared embarrassed, as though he'd been caught brow-beating the general's wife, for heaven's sake!

I remained in the chair. The doctor still didn't look up. He seemed to consider the interview over. Apparently he had finally learned some significant fact about me, some clue for which he had been probing.

What had I revealed? Did the doctor expect me to get up and leave without ever discussing Tony?

"Isn't it possible Tony is merely slow growing up? I can't believe something is wrong with him. I've watched every move he made this week. He seems to spend his time playing, like any child does. For instance, he spent this morning taking a flashlight apart and trying to pu—"

"He likes to take things apart, does he?" The doctor turned to look at Tony.

"Yes."

During the past half-hour, I had become so involved in the doctor's interrogation I had forgotten Tony. I looked at him now. He was watching the doctor gravely. The doctor bent over and spun his pen on the floor like a top. Tony stood observing the doctor's performance suspiciously.

"Couldn't he just be taking longer to mature?" I asked again. "Such a thing is possible, isn't it?"

He stared at Tony a few moments. The spinning pen hadn't seemed to effect Tony as the doctor expected. He picked it up and pocketed it in apparent disappointment.

"I wouldn't care to make a judgment on the matter," he said, turning his attention back to the medical records.

I got up and took Tony's hand. I was shaking, feeling as though I had fought off a physical assault. Tony and I managed to walk through the waiting room and the door of the clinic. I hadn't understood the doctor, and he seemed to ignore my questions. Never had I felt such bewildering inability to communicate. It was as though the doctor and I spoke different languages.

*   *   *

This was the first of many incomprehensible experiences. My husband and I were never actually told whether Tony's diagnosis was autistic, schizophrenic or "disturbed". In fact, no one would mention any of those terms for several years. Some doctors don't feel obligated to explain anything to patients, and perhaps our therapists decided their treatment would be most effective if the parents remained awed by the medical profession and ignorant about their child's diagnosis. I confess to having some bewildering thoughts and feelings about being abnormal during the next couple of years. I wasn't inclined to discuss them with a doctor or psychologist who knew something he wasn't telling me. However, even if I had found a therapist I trusted, I would have still preferred to work out my own solutions to any problems we may have had. Since I was unable to convince most people how strangely doctors were suddenly behaving, I wrote everything down, trying to capture every nuance and detail. I'd never had ambition to write anything, but I was desperate to make someone understand. Committing everything to paper was also a way to assure myself it was really happening. Eventually I discovered writing to be more therapeutic than any therapist could have been. If I hadn't happened upon this way to deal with my frustration, I probably wouldn't have remembered what Tony was like during those years. I wouldn't have remembered what I was like, for I would grow as much as Tony would.

CHAPTER 4

Is delayed speech "normal"?

The weeks after our second visit to the pediatrician, while awaiting Tony's appointment at the psychiatric clinic, were awful. My mind was in chaos. It was years before I achieved any understanding of that experience. Eventually I learned to describe it in an amusing manner, but I'd still find myself crying all over the typewriter.

I'd suffered the first real shock of my life. Ike was away. Much of the time I was alone with the children—and my thoughts. During the days I talked to neighbors, took care of the children and went on with my life. Night after night I lay awake pondering the pediatrician's bewildering cross-examination. I analyzed his every word, gesture and facial expression, again and again, trying to understand the purpose of his strange interrogation. What had he been trying to find out? What had he thought might be wrong with Tony? (About which he "wouldn't care to make a judgment".) He'd paid little attention to Tony. His concern seemed to be with me. He was looking for something wrong with me, some abnormality serious enough to effect Tony.

I'd never questioned my sanity. My parents had been blissfully ignorant about psychology, and I had never paid much attention to it.
"Suppressed hostilities", "inferiority complexes" and "emotional problems" might be cliches now, but meant little to me at that time. Before
talk shows, people didn't spend time discussing their feelings, and I
never knew anyone who worried about their self-esteem. The world
consisted of sane people and insane people, and no one had ever
expressed doubt that I was among the sane ones —until now.

One reason for my vulnerability to such fears was probably an aware-
ness of being a little different. For instance, I sometimes found it difficult to accept commonly held beliefs. At election time, I nearly always
voted for the loser. Sometimes I was unable to believe the most univer-
sally accepted scientific pronouncements. For example, evolution was
defined as "random mutation and survival of the fittest", but I could
never managed to believe the "random" part, regardless of how many
authorities stated it to be a "scientific fact". Also, my interests were often
not those of a typical woman. I rarely became excited about dresses,
hats, hair-do's, sterling silver, the color—or even the existence—of
kitchen curtains. I had other interests, but could Tony have inherited so
much of my divergent nature he regarded everything people did,
including talking, as not worth imitating? I'd never spent much energy
regretting my differences, and it had never before occurred to me one of
them might qualify me as abnormal.

The doctor and I hadn't discussed clothes or home decoration, I
reminded myself. Sometimes long, dark, sleepless nights I vowed to
phone the pediatrician and demand to know what mysterious information he had discovered about me. In the reality of daylight, I never mus-
tered the courage to contact that menacing doctor again, even on the
phone. I stayed home with the children and awaited the appointment at
the psychiatric clinic.

While I waited, sentences floated to the forefront of my mind, ideas I
had read or heard about somewhere, such as "a very intelligent child

who withdrew because his mother did not talk to him when he was a baby." That couldn't apply to Tony. I found talking to my babies natural.

There was something else I had heard once: "Children who are slow to talk sometimes grow up to be creative and exceptionally well-adjusted." I was confident all my children would grow up to be well adjusted. (I still hadn't realized parents aren't given the responsibility of creating their children—that most babies are already people when born—and parents have only limited power to alter them.)

I also remembered reading somewhere of a child (described by a psychologist as extremely intelligent) who wouldn't talk because he didn't have to; he pushed his mother around and got what he wanted. Tony pushed us. He pushed someone into the kitchen and up to the refrigerator when he was hungry. However, Tony didn't push us because he didn't want to talk; he didn't know how to talk.

I also remembered reading of a psychologist claiming, "An unusually intelligent child sometimes won't play with other children because he knows he is different." That sounded silly to say about any child, and in Tony's case, he didn't pay enough attention to other children to notice any differences.

One night it struck me all these remembered statements involved children with exceptional intelligence. I turned on the light, got out of bed and looked up genius in the encyclopedia. This authority stated some psychologists consider genius similar to a neurosis or psychosis, theorizing conflicts were channeled into productive pursuits instead of violent behavior. (That might sound silly, but it was in my encyclopedia, and I'm convinced some of psychology's present-day theories are no less nonsensical.)

I sat shivering on the floor by the bookcase, in my nightgown, with the encyclopedia in my lap. Could that be what the doctor thought was wrong with me? Did he suspect me of being a closet genius and believe Tony had inherited this "neurosis" or "psychosis" from me?

The subject of intelligence made me uncomfortable. I knew my IQ was probably above average, and I had a knack for mathematics and spatial relations. Nevertheless, I had enough sense to realize there was nothing remarkable about my intelligence as society usually defines the term. Yet I did have certain abilities (or lack of abilities) to an extreme, especially for a woman. (It would be years before neurologists began to discuss the difference between the analytical, masculine brain and the intuitive, feminine brain, but I'd often been aware I found men mentally, though not emotionally, easier to understand than women.) Women are often accused of "thinking with their emotions". Admittedly, I could become highly emotional, but I seemed able to recognize my feelings and could often think objectively in spite of them. More significantly, my inability to believe anything because I wanted to, or because everyone else believed it, had caused me to acquire some unorthodox opinions. Unorthodox ideas frighten many people, and I'd learned to keep mine to myself. My doubts about religion would have offended most of the people with whom I grew up. Never having spent much effort trying to analyze my abilities or lack of abilities, I vaguely thought of them as intelligence.

As a teen-aged girl, out-smarting boys at anything hadn't felt particularly advantageous. Playing dumb seemed expedient, and I enjoyed clowning. In the architecture building at the university a big tub of water was used to soak art paper before taping it to drawing boards. Architecture students were notorious for such juvenile pranks as dropping bags of water out the window onto unsuspecting victims. I was the only girl in my class, and in 1940 it was considered unladylike for girls to wear trousers. My classmates threw me in that tub of water whenever I appeared at school in slacks. They claimed such dunking was traditional. In retaliation, I talked someone into helping me dismantle their desks and reassemble them on the roof. Another time they locked me in the phone booth for several hours and fed me Coca Cola by a straw through the keyhole. I was unable to keep from laughing. The truth

was, I enjoyed being the victim of pranks as much as I delighted in playing them. Architecture was really my minor. I was majoring in fun.

Now, as I pondered my "abnormality", I remembered another incident at the university. Traditionally, students stayed up together and
worked all night before turning in their designs. We called it being *en
charette*, a term borrowed from French architecture students who continued to work on their projects after they were placed "on the cart".
One such evening, I finished my work early and lay down on a couch to
take a nap. Several of the boys were talking in a foreign language. They
switched to English, and I realized their discussion wasn't meant for my
ears. While I lay there lay there wondering how to avoid being caught
eavesdropping, one boy asked,

"Do you suppose she's actually asleep over there?"

"You can never tell about that wacky female," another boy commented. "She's not as dumb as she acts, you know."

I'd nearly choked to keep from laughing out loud. The boy was a
friend. If he'd found me out, he didn't seem to hold it against me. Now,
I suddenly wondered if that boy's remark could have more ominous significance. The pediatrician had also detected my abnormality and
seemed to believe it had damaged Tony. I felt overwhelmed with shame
and humiliation, thinking of all the people who must have noticed my
deviation while I sailed through life oblivious to the glaring defect. Such
a flaw might be overlooked in someone who accomplishes something,
but I'd neglected to produce anything that might be considered the
result of genius. The pediatrician had even unearthed my embarrassing
secret by using my own private IQ test: agnosticism. Ridiculous as it
now sounds, I assumed agnosticism was a sure measure of intelligence.

If I was ever an atheist, it was only briefly. Atheists are confident anything that science cannot explain does not exist, while agnostics are not
certain about much of anything. However, at that time I didn't attach
much importance to the distinction between the two. Part of my suffering
over my "genius psychosis" may have been a reluctance to acknowledge the

intolerant absurdity of my "IQ test". Today as more myths and legends of traditional religions are being questioned, some "scientifically minded" materialists seem to regard their newfound atheism a "profound truth". (Sort of like the heady experience of discovering there is no Santa Claus. Boy, were those kids dumb who still believed that hoax!) Perhaps people are often tempted to regard anyone who disagrees with them of lesser in intelligence, but twentieth century materialists have somehow managed to even intimidate people who aren't materialists into regarding belief in scientific materialism as a sign of intelligence. (One wonders what was so intelligent about belief in Marxism, eugenics, reductionism, Freudian analysis, sociobiology, Neo-Darwinism, the notion that free will doesn't really exist—or the many other the fads espoused by this "intellectual elite"?) The pediatrician may have using such an "IQ test". Or, on the other hand, he may have been merely trying to find out if I was Jewish. I've read Jewish children are susceptible to emotional problems. However Jewish people were heavily represented in psychiatric professions and may have simply been more inclined to send their kids to psychiatrists. Such thoughts were in the future, though, and at that time my "genius psychosis" was excruciatingly painful.

One night as I lay in bed brooding over my aberrations and what they had done to Tony, I found myself giggling. I remembered the time I wrote two checks for twenty dollars each because I couldn't remember how to spell forty. Also, there was the time I had to postpone writing to my sister because I couldn't remember her married name.

Some genius!

My sense of humor was returning, and without understanding them, I managed to push those disturbing thoughts from my mind.

When I emerged from my agonizing self-examination, I began to seek opportunities for Tony to be with other children. I took him to Sunday school. Marching around the nursery with the three year olds, singing Onward *Christian Soldiers*, I tried to make it look like fun. Tony remained unconvinced. He was only interested in opening the piano or finding out what was in the broom closet. He didn't seem frightened of the other children. He glanced curiously at them a couple of times, while they sang and recited verses, as though wondering what they were doing—and why. Finally Tony got out of his little chair and lay down on the floor. The other children gathered around and asked what Tony was doing—and why.

I watched Tony constantly. He became suspicious and refused to do anything under my scrutiny. I coaxed him into repeating some words one afternoon, but when I tried again the next day, Tony took himself indignantly into his room and slammed the door. Efforts to persuade him to learn anything seemed futile.

One day I found Tony on top of some boxes stacked on a chair trying to knock a box of cookies off a high shelf with a broom. Tony's reactions were fast, and his expression was bright-eyed and alert. Most of his mischief seemed to require imagination. Tony, then, could not be mentally retarded. If he wasn't unhappy—didn't have an emotional problem— what else might be wrong with him?

∗   ∗   ∗

When the day arrived for our appointment at the psychiatric clinic, much of my fear had faded. That pediatrician was not an authority on emotional problems. On the other hand, a scientifically trained professional at a psychiatric clinic would quickly see Tony was not unhappy. Confident such specialists understood human emotions, and could fix any that were out of kilter, I finally spoke to a psychologist at Letterman Hospital Psychiatric Clinic. He was an agreeable young man who introduced himself as Dr. Berger. Tony, probably sensing men in white coats upset Mommy, sat quietly on my lap and gravely watched the doctor instead of looking for something to dismantle. "What seems to be the trouble with your child?" the doctor asked.

"I don't believe anything is wrong with him. He doesn't talk much and is still in diapers, but so was my other son until the age of three." The pediatrician had appeared to consider it significant that Tony took things apart, and I continued, "He takes the knobs off the T.V., unscrews pieces off the sewing machine, and clocks seem to disintegrate faster than we can buy them."

"Not so fast!" he said, trying to write everything down.

"Tony has temper tantrums. I've never discovered an effective way to deal with tantrums, so I ignore them."

He nodded in seeming approval.

"Someone once suggested throwing a glass of water at him. My two older children thought that sounded like fun, and I tried it. Tony grabbed the glass out of my hand and threw it back at me. Then he continued his tantrum."

The psychologist—still writing furiously—smiled understandingly.

"One morning Tony wanted outside and couldn't get the door open. He got a hammer and broke the glass out of it. When I scolded him, I could see by his puzzled expression he didn't know what the fuss was about."

Although shocked when Tony bashed in that glass, I had recently decided he at least showed intelligence by figuring out how to get through a locked door. Undoubtedly the psychologist, who was an authority on intelligence, would agree.

"Would you say reward and punishment are methods which work with this child?" he asked.

"No!"

He grinned. "You sound as though you speak from experience."

I nodded ruefully, and he continued.

"Do you remember anything unusual about Tony as a baby?"

"No. He was a cute baby. He did get sick once. The doctors suspected asthma. Tony recovered when I stopped forcing him to eat solid foods."

When my first child was born, the medical profession had decided tiny infants should be introduced to baby-food. My first son had resisted with an effective defense: he passed out at the feel of a spoon on his lips. My infant daughter was less defiant and ended up in the hospital with diarrhea. I still made an effort to obey doctors' orders and force food into Tony's mouth. When I suggested to my pediatrician food might be causing Tony's asthmatic reaction, he had recommended I experiment to discover which food. Although feeling guilty about disobeying a doctor, I was reluctant to experiment. I never gave Tony another bite until he became old enough to put food into his own mouth. Since then he'd been so healthy he'd rarely seen a doctor.

"Now," the doctor said, putting more paper on his clipboard, "Let's get some information about you."

"What do you want to know?" I shot back. It sounded louder than I intended. "I mean, oh well—"

I had been bracing myself for that question, and my defensive reaction was apparent. I took a deep breath and, struggling to sound calm and composed, managed to regain control of myself. I inquired with a gracious smile and unconcerned serenity,

"What would you like to know about me?"

The psychologist suppressed a smile. Perhaps the pediatrician who made the appointment had warned him about my reaction to that line of questioning.

"Just a little background material," he said.

"I grew up in Ukiah, went to the university, went to Alaska, got married—"

"Wait a minute! Let's start over and go more slowly."

Then he asked a few questions that didn't feel at all like the pediatrician's interrogation. As I had sensed the pediatrician believed I was concealing something, I soon felt this psychologist had already reached the conclusion I was well adjusted and emotionally mature. His questions seemed for the purpose of verifying my emotional stability. Tony slid off my lap to close a cabinet drawer.

"Were you and your husband getting along when Tony was born?"

"Well, my husband and I have had our disagreements, like all married people, but—"

"But you weren't about to split up, or anything?"

"Oh no." My unplanned pregnancy had been a stressful time for us, but we never considered separating.

"You attended the University of California," he continued, looking over his notes. "Where did you live while you were in college?"

"I shared an apartment with three other girls."

"You had the same roommates all through college?"

"Yes. Twenty years later, we are still close friends."

I recognized the point of his clever question. He must realize emotionally unstable people might have trouble maintaining long-term relationships. Tony had apparently decided this white-coat-clad man was not threatening Mommy. Losing interest in the psychologist, Tony was crawling under the desk.

"Did you graduate from Cal.?"

"No."

"Oh? Why not?"

"I changed majors several times. When the war began, I went to work in the shipyards."

"Then you went to Alaska. Why did you go up there?"

I looked at him blankly. Eighteen years ago no one had seemed to think I needed a reason.

"I don't know. Just for fun, I guess."

He appeared to find the answer acceptable, and asked about Ike's rank in the army when we were married.

"He was a lieutenant…"

I glanced around the office. I was looking for the psychologist's coat with some gold bars on it, so I could say, "that kind". I finally said,

"Oh, that bottom kind. You know, that bottom kind."

It had always confused me one became a second lieutenant before becoming a first lieutenant, *but dammit, why had I said something stupid like that?* Dr. Berger was suppressing another smile and didn't appear to consider my lapse serious. (As I talked to more psychologists during the next few years, I was always tense. I strove to sound normal and casual, never intending to make jokes. Yet I often heard myself utter something preposterous. Certainly, becoming so relaxed I forgot my husband's rank was ridiculous.)

"Let's find out something about your husband," the doctor said. "Did he go to college?"

"No."

"Oh? Do you know why not?"

"I'm not sure. I think he only wanted to work on a newspaper."

The psychologist asked about Ike's father, who was an eye surgeon. He seemed interested in Ike's grandfather, and the book Ike's father wrote about him.

"What about your father?" Dr. Berger asked.

I hesitated. I could mention Daddy's inventions. That would be in the spirit of all this interest in our superior intellects.

Then I stopped myself. Depicting Daddy as a brilliant, but unsuccessful inventor would be a bit of an exaggeration.

"He was a automobile mechanic," I answered.

Tony had plenty of relatives who were grade-school dropouts, which wasn't considered so disgraceful a few generations ago. I suspected such ancestors wouldn't interest Dr. Berger though, and didn't mention them.

The psychologist appeared to have run out of questions.

"Doesn't an emotional problem imply some unhappiness?" I asked.

"Not necessarily. Sometimes a child might feel guilty about something he doesn't understand, such as a car accident."

I struggled daily to persuade Tony to feel guilty about the things he did, such as throwing the cat out the window or smashing holes in the walls. Before we nailed barricades over his window, Tony once threw all his clothes, bedding and toys out on to the street below. So far I'd been unable to evoke the least sign of remorse for anything the little rascal did. I couldn't imagine Tony suffering guilt over something for which he wasn't responsible.

"Do you have any more questions?" Dr. Berger asked.

"Just one, and I suppose you won't answer it: Do you think anything is wrong with Tony?"

"No, I can't answer that now," he replied as he sat watching Tony dismantle a mechanical pencil he'd found under the desk. "We don't th—I mean we *hope* nothing is wrong with your son. But we'll have to wait for an evaluation."

I nodded, and the psychologist added, "In any case, it might be interesting to see exactly what kind of a child you have here!"

His tone was optimistic, almost excited. At that time, many psychologists believed autistic children—despite their retarded level of functioning—were actually extremely intelligent. (That says something about their ability to measure intelligence, doesn't it?) Although I had never heard of autism, this psychologist seemed to act as though he suspected our whole family of being awfully smart. He hadn't asked if we graduated from college; he asked why we didn't. Remembering the horror of thinking something was wrong with me, I tried to resist another attack of "genius psychosis". Nevertheless, by the time I left, I'd had a relapse. This time my psychosis wasn't painful; it was a heady, lofty feeling. I felt confidently qualified to offer my opinion on any subject. Perhaps I should make another effort to understand relativity—or maybe even quantum mechanics.

Dr. Berger suggested we walk down to the end of the hall to allow Tony to become familiar with the playroom where the evaluation would take place. I'm sure poor little Tony believed something frightening and terrible was about to happen to him. Mommy seemed convinced of it lately. He took one look at that room full of "little-people equipment" and decided this might be where it would happen. He charged into me and knocked me out of the room. Then he got behind and pushed me down the long hall, through the waiting room full of people, and out of the building. Most of my attention was on coping with Tony. Nevertheless, I left with an impression of the psychologist watching with an amused look on his face. Surely no one would regard the tragedy of an abnormal child with amusement. The psychologist would look more somber if he thought Tony were retarded, wouldn't he?

*   *   *

The psychiatric clinic had a long waiting list, and our appointment for Tony's evaluation was not for several months. Determined to learn what psychology was about, I got a pile of books from the library. Psychoanalysts seemed inclined to take simple, often silly, ideas and mesmerize their readers with obscure, verbose technical language. I became so entangled in their recondite, multi-vocal structures of circumlocutory, obscure macabre, cryptographic polysyllabification and tangled esoteric, elliptic, hyperbolic hypotheses and postulates, that like my infant son at the feel of a spoon on his lips, my mind tried to escape into unconsciousness. (I later heard of parents being told their autistic child suffered from Symbiotic Parasitic Infantile Psychosis.) I read that Freud, the father of psychoanalysis, hadn't considered mother important in a boy's life. He blamed most male emotional problems on an *Oedipus Complex*, a suppressed, guilt-laden wish to murder father and ravish mother. Freud claimed little girls are obsessed by envy of their fathers' penis and feel castrated. (Some men sure have an exaggerated view of the esthetic qualities of that piece of anatomy!) Freud's definition of a *neurotic* seemed to be anyone suffering confusion about what they thought or felt. He claimed an effective therapist must himself have suffered such painful befuddlement, and undergone analysis, in order to understand his patients. A couple of colleagues, Jung and Adler, while remaining faithful to psychoanalysis, disagreed with Freud's emphasis on infantile sex. Freud and his followers suffered anguish and emotional trauma over Jung's treachery and Adler's betrayal.

Years later, I would read of another of Freud's theories, one about a direct connection between women's noses and their wombs. He made this scientific discovery when he learned he could treat menstrual cramps by applying cocaine to a woman's nose. Freud and a colleague operated on women's noses to treat hysteria, which was thought to take place in the womb. Being inexperienced surgeons, they nearly killed one woman by leaving a length of gauze in her nose. Many of Freud's worst blunders were kept concealed from the public for many years by his devoted disciples, whose belief in psychoanalysis resembled a religious commitment.

I turned to more general psychology books, where I found more nonsense For instance, I read navy frogmen fear women, and find in the sea the security of their mother's womb. In an old psychology book I found a description of a "withdrawn" child whose symptoms might have resembled Tony's. The psychologist who "cured" him discovered the child was in the care of a woman with a low IQ who talked too much. The psychologist felt the child, who had a high IQ, withdrew because of aversion to so much lowbrow chatter. Here was another "withdrawn" child who had turned out to be exceptionally intelligent. This must be the diagnosis Dr. Berger suspected for Tony. Dr. Berger must be aware these children didn't "withdraw". Psychologists must have finally realized late development was natural for some highly intelligent children.

As the months passed I worried less about Tony. My other two children didn't seem concerned. Sherry boosted my confidence with some of her own distinctive brand of logic.

"Well really, Mother," she said. "I know why Tony didn't grow up. You never let him have his birthdays."

She was about to become seven and knew it couldn't possibly be accomplished without a party. Ike arrived home from Greenland, worried, but reassured to see Tony looking bright eyed and healthy as ever. Tony was still unpredictable. He got up early one morning to fix his own breakfast, beating a dozen eggs all over the living room rug. Ike took him to town, and was startled when Tony lay down on his stomach and drank out of the gutter.

"Drinking out of the gutter might be unsanitary," I assured Ike, "but it shows more intelligence than standing and crying that he's thirsty."

We resumed the busy, satisfying life of a suburban family with small children. I awaited Tony's evaluation, smugly expecting to be informed we were the parents of a gifted child. At that time I hadn't questioned the twentieth century notion that IQ and academic performance were valid measures of a gifted child. Today I might attach more importance to other traits, such as instincts, perseverance, personality, character, courage, responsibility, sensitivity, intuition or creativity. Science still hasn't learned to measure such traits. Nevertheless many people regard them as "real".

CHAPTER 5

What do psychological tests measure?

The date for Tony's psychiatric evaluation finally arrived. Everyone seemed to regard psychology with awe, and I saw no reason to doubt its validity. Much of what I'd read in the psychology books seemed silly, but the books were probably obsolete. Remembering Dr. Berger's insightful questions, I assumed the science had become more precise. Earlier ideas about the human psyche might have included superstitions and delusions, but modern psychologists employed scientific methods, didn't they? Ike and I arrived at the clinic with Tony and sat in the waiting room. While retrieving Tony from crawling under—or on top of—the reception desk, I cautiously observed people in adjacent chairs, speculating what mysterious cures and information they might be seeking from these technical experts. A tall young man with expressive, brown eyes came out and shyly introduced himself as Dr. Lavalle. I'd expected to see Dr. Berger, but Dr. Lavalle was pleasant and seemed to convey interested concern.

To our surprise, Dr. Lavalle asked Ike and me to take some tests ourselves while he examined Tony. Ike complied with good-natured curiosity. Military families often obey without asking questions. However Tony had no desire to go into that room full of "little people equipment" and have his intelligence measured and he objected when I left. I stood anxiously out in the hall listening to him cry. These psychologists were the latest authorities on what was good for children. I did want to trust such experts and forced myself not to interfere. Finally Dr. Lavalle came out and asked me to remain in the playroom.

Tony found some blocks and began to make a train. The psychologist sat silently and watched him. I sat silently and watched the psychologist. Awed by this mysterious scientific process, I wondered what inscrutable method he was using to measure Tony's intelligence.

After Dr. Lavalle observed Tony for an hour, he asked us to return the next day. This time Ike stayed in the playroom with Tony, and I took the tests Ike had taken the day before, the details of which we had been warned not to discuss.

From a stack of cards with enigmatic phrases on them, I was told to pick twenty that applied to me, putting them in order with the most descriptive on top. From another stack of identical cards, I picked twenty to describe Ike and Tony. Finally I selected cards I *wished* applied to me, and ones I wished described Ike and Tony.

Most of the cards bore familiar words, but when presented out of context like that, I found their meanings elusive. *Modest*, for instance, probably didn't mean wearing enough clothes in public. Even after looking up the word in a dictionary I sometimes ponder its meaning. If a person has a "modest estimate of his abilities", but the abilities are even more modest than the estimate, does the term still apply? The whole thing seemed difficult to determine. In any case, my recent genius psychosis hardly entitled me to claim that one, and I ignored it.

Did being a Cub Scout Den Mother qualify me to use *leader*? Probably not. I wasn't even a very good Den Mother. Guy, who was usually cooperative, became as uncontrollable as the rest of those rowdy little nine- year-old boys. They spent more time on top of the house and up in trees than doing the projects suggested in the Cub Scout manual.

Warm surely didn't mean temperature, but come to think of it, what did it mean? *Cold* must be the opposite, whatever it meant. *Hot* and *cool* seemed to be missing. The harder I tried to figure out exact meanings, the more confused I became.

Maybe I should stop doing so much thinking. I'd let my subconscious make selections. Surely it was my subconscious that concerned these psychologists. I did it rather playfully, never dreaming those silly cards could get us into trouble. Dr. Berger had appeared to have a sense of humor, and I could probably think of some explanation for any choice he might question.

Clinging vine didn't appeal to me, but *independent* and *self-reliant* sounded fine, and I put them on top of descriptions of each of us. I rarely disliked anyone, but to be honest, some people bored me. I chose can *be indifferent to others* for all of us. It certainly described Tony, and I felt an impulse to defend my child's personality.

Twenty cards for each stack were hard to find. Many sounded unflattering, such as *stern but fair, believes everything they are told,* and *generous to a fault.* (I took their word that generosity could actually be a fault.)

Then I tried to pick cards I wished applied. I wasn't actually dissatisfied with any of us. Everyone, including Tony, was entitled to be content with their own nature. But since this was a sort of game, maybe I should try to upgrade us all a little. I wished Tony were more precocious, but there was no card for that. None of those cards felt like an improvement. Finally, I threw in one called *smug and self-satisfied.* Perhaps we all had more self-esteem than was justified. Incredible as it now seems, I believed psychologists could measure our innermost natures from that scientific test.

When we finished, Dr. Lavalle promised someone would phone when they reached a conclusion about Tony. When we got home, I told Tony to go wash his face. Tony rarely paid attention when we told him to do things, but this time he startled us.

"Go bye-bye car?"

"Why no, dear! We are going to eat dinner."

"I talk," coaxed Tony. "One, two, free, four, five. I talk."

"Did you hear that?" I exclaimed, grabbing Tony up in a gleeful hug,

"Maybe he's thinking he would have talked before if he'd know it was all this important to us," Ike suggested. Guy and Sherry laughed with us. Tony seemed to tolerate our jubilation indulgently. More than a week passed before someone called from the psychiatric clinic.

"Could you come in tomorrow and talk to Dr. Dingle?"

"Shall we bring Tony?" I asked, wondering who Dr. Dingle was.

"No. The appointment is for you."

"Do you mean my husband shouldn't come either?"

"No."

Was there something more than merely telling us there was nothing wrong with Tony? But if something was wrong, why had they sent for me to come alone? And why wasn't Dr. Berger or Dr. Lavalle to reveal the results of the examination? I must have fouled up those damned cards! *I should have taken them more seriously.* I'd expected my nightmare to end when the medical profession finally examined Tony and pronounced him normal. I shed some tears of fear, frustration and disappointment.

With foreboding, I met Dr. Dingle at the psychiatric clinic the next day. He turned out to be a plump, eager looking young man with a round, cheerful face and a smooth, pink complexion—an adult sized cherub. I followed him down the hall to his office, and seated myself uneasily across the desk from him. He explained he was organizing a group of women who would meet once a week for a year. While their children were receiving therapy, the mothers would discuss their similar family problems.

"Family problems!" I exclaimed. "I don't have any family problems I want to discuss with anyone."

"Well then, you aren't yet aware of your problems." (That was an understatement.)

"But, what's wrong with Tony?"

"We don't know."

Oh hell! He wasn't going to tell me Tony was one of those highly intelligent "withdrawn" children I'd read of in the psychology books.

"Then how do you know something is wrong with him?" I argued. "I've heard of several children who didn't talk until they were four and grew up to be fine people."

"It isn't only that Tony doesn't talk. His symptoms are globular."

He probably meant global. Sounded pompous to me.

"Tony's older brother was slow to talk, and he is a very intelligent child."

"Now, there is no denying Tony is a very, very bright little boy," the psychologist said. "But intelligence has abs-o-lutely nothing to do with this."

"If you think some problem in our family is causing Tony to be the way he is, you are abs-o-lutely wrong."

"We'll see," he muttered.

"I tell you there isn't. Don't you believe me?'

"Yes, we believe you." (He obviously didn't.) "Nevertheless, I urge you to try the group for a few weeks." Then he mumbled under his breath, "We'll see if we can't get a little transference going here."

I had come across that word in the psychology books. Psychiatric patients often transfer their feelings of love or hatred from their parents to the therapist, and female patients "fall in love" with their analyst. Did therapists come right out and suggest such a thing? I stared at him in horror.

"I mean, it's about time we get Tony to show some emotion," Dr. Dingle added hastily.

I'd read the term also might refer to the transference, at a certain age, of a child's affection from his mother to his father. Maybe that's what he meant. But what was that mysterious diagnosis Dr. Berger seemed to have in mind when he said, "It might be interesting to see exactly what kind of a child we have here!"? I tried to repeat some of the things I'd told the other psychologist, probably sounding more desperate than coherent.

"But the things he took apart?"

"Tony takes things apart?"

"And drinking out of the gutter."

"He drinks out of the gutter?"

"And bashing in the front door, I mean, and the other children, ignoring them that is, and pulling up the neighbor's flowers. It was like the things he makes with blocks. Besides! I just remembered! Tony talks. He told us so. One, two, free, four, five. I talk."

The psychologist was eyeing me dubiously.

I needed to stop raving and try to regain some composure.

"I don't mean to sound ungrateful," I said, falling back in my chair and trying to relax. "By offering me therapy, you are trying to do me a service. I appreciate your concern. But—"

"Bring Tony in next week to get acquainted with Dr. Lavalle. He's the psychologist who will work with Tony." Dr. Dingle's face dimpled with a smile, as he got up to open the door for me. "You'll be surprised at the progress Tony will make with our help."

I hadn't meant I was so grateful for his good intentions I wanted psychotherapy. However the psychologist seemed determined to administer some, whether I wanted it or not. I left his office, dazed, and with a premonition something disastrous had happened, and met Dr. Berger in the hall.

"Hi," he greeted me. "Was your little boy ever evaluated?"

"Yes," I answered glumly.

"How is everything?"

I didn't answer. I figured he was in a better position than I to know "how everything is" around this place.

    *   *   *

When I returned to the clinic with Tony the following week, both psychologists, Dr. Lavalle and Dr. Dingle, met us in the waiting room. There was something different about their attitudes. I didn't know about the controversy over autism raging in the medical world, and was unaware that proponents of various theories were jealously competing to prove their hypotheses. However, long before I ever heard of autism, I often sensed some doctors viewed Tony as a rare, interesting case. I sensed it that afternoon. I decided these two psychologists must have finally compared notes with Dr. Berger. They probably now realized "exactly what kind of a child we had here"—whatever kind that was. We walked down to the playroom. Tony remembered where the blocks were kept and began to make an airplane.

"Does he spend a lot of time playing with blocks?" Dr. Lavalle asked with a hint of excitement.

"Yes. Some of his creations are elaborate and quite beautiful."

I had learned principles of artistic design while studying architecture. However no one had taught Tony; he seemed to have been born with such knowledge. Tony was purposefully arranging the blocks.

"Note his use of symmetry," Dr. Lavalle said to Dr. Dingle.

Dr. Dingle didn't respond.

"Did you note his use of symmetry?" Dr. Lavalle repeated.

"Hmph," Dr. Dingle grunted, with an uneasy glance toward me.

Did he feel such technical, psychological matters shouldn't be discussed in front of uninformed laymen, such as mothers?

"Let's go down to my office and have a little chat," Dr. Dingle said to me.

Tony, busy with the blocks, didn't object to me leaving. I walked down the hall with Dr. Dingle. *Damn! Another psychiatric interrogation!* How did this psychologist come up with the bizarre notion these psychiatric inquisitions could be considered "little chats"? How did I ever get into this ridiculous predicament, anyway? Most people live their entire lives without having their sanity or emotional stability questioned.

Dr. Dingle opened his office door for me. I glanced furtively around the room. Thank heavens there didn't seem to be any couches. I sat on the edge of a chair and clutched my purse in my lap.

"Now," Dr. Dingle began, as he sat back comfortably and crossed his chubby legs. "Tell me about yourself."

"That corny question again!"

"Well then, " he persisted, "what sort of things do you enjoy doing?"

"Yesterday I stopped at a railroad crossing with the children in the car. My daughter asked, Mommy, did you ever drive a choo-choo train?' I remembered the night I drove the *Nancy Hanks* from Atlanta to Savannah, tooting the whistle like mad. That was sort of fun."

The story wasn't a complete fabrication. I'd met a vice president of the railroad in the club car. He invited me up into the engine, to sit in the driver's seat and pull the whistle a few times. However, I realized I'd fouled up again—I'd said something flippant. But why should I have to convince this psychologist I was normal? Such a task seemed hopeless, like proving a negative. I looked him in the eye, mentally daring him to make something out of my remark.

"What else do you enjoy?" He was trying not to smile, apparently not wishing to encourage levity.

"I garden, play Tournament Bridge, and read a lot. I've always managed to find something to keep busy and happy." At the moment I probably wasn't presenting a convincing picture of a woman who enjoys life.

"What type of things do you *not* enjoy?"

Oh, cocktail parties, women's luncheons." I could have added, "and psychologists asking impertinent questions,"—but didn't.

He sat and looked at me a few moments. "Tell me about your childhood," he said.

How could anyone sit and so cheerfully display such unmitigated gall?

"Tell me about your childhood," he repeated.

I continued to glare at him, but his gaze didn't waver.

"My father was an alcoholic," I finally said. "That is supposed to suggest an unhappy childhood, I imagine, but mine was not. I seem to have a talent for enjoying life, and I enjoyed life as a child, in spite of a sometimes hectic home life."

I was capable of lying, but not when taken by surprise like that. Besides, it would probably be futile to lie to psychologists; they had scientific methods of uncovering the truth, didn't they? My father's drinking wasn't a deep, dark secret. Many people in the town where I grew up were probably aware of it. Most people had enough manners not to bring up the subject, but psychologists apparently weren't shy about asking outrageous questions. Dr. Dingle finally seemed to become aware of my anger, and changed the subject.

"How do you feel about coming to group therapy?" he asked.

"A year would be a long time to sit and listen to the same women's problems."

"Yes, but after you become interested, you'll enjoy it. While you are in the group, Tony will be in the playroom with Dr. Lavalle. Allowing Tony to form a relationship with someone outside the family would be a good idea. That's the only reason for you to attend the group," he emphasized.

I realized it would be nice for Tony to have a friend. Tony ignored people. He wasn't so much unfriendly as uninterested, and his indifference soon discouraged everyone who tried to approach him. Psychiatry had never interested me. Nevertheless, although I had only a vague understanding of psychoanalysis, from the moment that pediatrician said "tell me about yourself", I sensed I would not enjoy psychotherapy.

*   *   *

Psychotherapy was a proposal for "fixing" psyches. Psychology was striving for status as part of materialistic science. Materialism regards people as complex machines, with a brain resembling a computer. Instincts are regarded as part of our genetic make up (hardware), but knowledge (software) is claimed to be the result of whatever is learned or experienced after birth. Free will has no place in a machine, and most materialists claim free will is an illusion. They argue that what we mistakenly suppose is free will is merely the inevitable result of molecules and neural connections in the brain. Mathematics is the language of science, and much of psychology was based upon statistics. Psychologists believed everyone was born "normal" (average). Faulty software (traumatic experiences) was thought to be responsible for those psyches falling outside the statistical average. I began to wonder if scientific studies had ever been conducted to determine whether a traumatic childhood actually produced neurotic adults. Psychiatric patients might report such a childhood because that was what the therapists expected. Others might allow themselves to be talked into remembering such damage for the weird reason that they enjoyed playing the role of victim. In any case I was an individual, not a statistic. I'd never had any trouble convincing people I didn't fit the statistical generalization about boys being better than girls at math. Surely after he got to know me, Dr. Dingle would soon realize I was not emotionally damaged by a traumatic childhood, and didn't need "fixing". However, in spite of my growing suspicion of psychotherapy, I was too much under the influence of "modern science" to deny Tony treatment the medical profession was insisting he must have. This, I had found myself agreeing to join Dr. Dingle's group.

CHAPTER 6

Should "normal" be equated with average?

Today it has become fashionable for psychiatry to declare clinical depression to be caused by "chemical imbalances". (Although no one has specified exactly which chemicals might be involved.) If these elusive chemicals were ever identified, I'm confident I'd prove to be blessed (or plagued) with an excess of whatever chemicals might prevent depression. Nevertheless, in 1961 all depression was thought to be the result of "damaged psyches". Ike and I had problems, but I was confident they hadn't affected Tony. Feeling no desire to discuss any of my problems with a psychologist, I had no intention of discussing Ike's.

I knew Freud had convinced everyone they were inhabited by something called a subconscious. This mysterious entity supposedly had a tendency to think naughty thoughts, but kept them a secret from our conscious selves. Sometimes this naughty subconscious took over and controlled our actions—without our knowledge or permission. It was believed that if one lay on a couch and talked, and a psychiatrist listened, the subconscious might be tricked into revealing itself. Once it was skillfully enticed out into the open by a therapist, the subconscious supposedly lost its power to control people's actions. (Not many people believe in Freudianism today, but in 1961, questioning such esoteric theories was as frowned upon as questioning Darwinism is today. People of the twentieth century would believe anything if it was so complicated they couldn't understand it, and if it was labeled "scientific".) In any case, if some people claimed to have a painful, hidden, complex, tortuous, broiling subconscious, I'd take their word for it. My emotions were seldom difficult for me to understand, and I was quite aware of my naughty thoughts. Nevertheless, I was convinced I was as normal as any neurotic, even if I lacked a subconscious.

There may be a flip side to being a "simple soul", as there might be for most human traits. Perhaps a measure of neurosis, or at least some conflict, is essential for understanding art and poetry, abilities to which I confessed a dismal lack. Symbolism seems important in art, and symbolic meanings eluded me. I couldn't resist wondering why poets don't simply say what they mean, instead of concealing it in symbolism. But while an inability to appreciate esoteric verse should be no cause for pride, I hardly regarded it pathological.

I remembered the excitement with which I left Ukiah at the age of eighteen, and boarded a Greyhound bus for the university. A friend had arranged for me to spend one night with her aunt in San Francisco. In possession of fifty dollars, which I'd saved, and carrying a suitcase full of my belongings, I arrived in Berkeley early the next morning. Before registering for classes, I located the campus employment office, where I obtained a job helping with the children and household chores in the home of a professor. To my dismay, the job didn't start until the next day, and I was left with the problem of where to spend that night.

I'd never been in a hotel. In fact, I was under the impression there was something unsavory about them. People made whispered comments about a woman in Ukiah who hung around the hotel. I was reluctant to take the ferry back to San Francisco for another night with the friend's aunt. An academic advisor was assigned to each enrolling freshman. Mine was probably puzzled by my aversion to hotels, but offered me the bed of her roommate, who wasn't expected until the next day. We saw no reason to inform the housemother.

The roommate arrived unexpectedly in the middle of the night. The housemother was exasperated to find an uninvited guest. Muttering to herself, she gave me a pillow and blanket and allowed me to sleep on a couch. It was an unsatisfactory beginning for my glorious adventure, but at least I hadn't had to brave the mysterious dangers of a hotel. The next day I moved into the professor's home. After paying my tuition (twenty-six dollars!), I blew the rest of my fifty dollars on clothes, including a pair of shoes with heels so high I could hardly balance myself on them.

My first months in Berkeley were spent in a euphoric haze of blissful excitement. During my childhood I'd wished my family were more like those described in movies and magazines. Now suddenly my parents were far away, and I was free to invent any kind of family I wished. I made my first friend because my name was Starke and hers was Stahl. Seated alphabetically in freshman classes, I helped Kay Stahl with math. The similar spelling of our names was the beginning of a friendship that would last for more than half a century. Soon we met Alice, a spunky sixteen-year-old orphan who had been earning her own living while still in high school. Then Phyllis joined us. We all lacked sophistication, even for our ages, but shared a sense of humor and enthusiasm for life.

During my second year in college, the four of us excitedly squeezed our meager possessions into a tiny studio apartment. We supported ourselves on about six dollars a week by working as waitresses and theater usherettes. We ate canned tuna, peanut butter and fresh vegetables, food which cost only pennies in those days. Coca Cola cost a nickel, so we drank water—but so did most people during the Depression. Kay owned a black velvet dress, which we all borrowed for special dates. We were usually able to scrape up a quarter for an occasional hot fudge Sunday or a trip to San Francisco on the bus. We discovered credit. Buying clothes in a department store, we contracted to pay for them at fifty cents a week. The clothes wore out before that account was paid off, leaving me with a life-long aversion to credit.

Because math was easy for me, I choose that as my major. My thinking ran along analytical lines, and an understanding of people did not come easy to me. Today, people are no longer such a baffling mystery, and I think most of that insight was achieved from books. One summer while still in high school I had decided to read every volume in the Ukiah library - alphabetically. I finish the A's, which included Jane Austin and Louisa May Alcott, but the B's turned out to contain some pretty weird tales, and I abandoned the project. In any case, when I started college, I was hardly aware of my own feelings or beliefs, and had no idea what went on in other people's heads. As a result, I was sometimes agonizingly shy around strangers. Nevertheless, shy does not necessarily mean timid. I determinedly confronted strange situations, and approached strangers, even when trembling with nervous fear.

Curiosity attracted us to the foreign students at the university, but we also made friends where we worked, which included cooks, waitresses, firefighters and baseball players. We worked and attended classes—but we also found time and energy to swim, ice skate, ride horseback, go camping, and attend parties and dances. We stayed up all night with anyone willing to talk, trying to discuss our newly found world of ideas.

For me, fun—and the discovery of this big exciting world—took precedence over the pursuit of a career. One day I wondered what one might actually do after becoming a mathematician—other than teach, which didn't appeal to me. (I always hated telling other people what to do, not a valuable trait for a teacher.) I consulted an academic counselor, who suggested mathematicians might be statisticians—whatever they did. I changed my major to art. My drawing skills were adequate, and while I never really understood art, I liked artists. When Pearl Harbor was bombed, I had switched majors again and was studying architecture, which combined my drawing and mathematical skills.

When the war started, I quit school and went to work in the drafting department at a shipyard. There, besides indulging in my fondness for pranks and jokes, I tried to interest friends in buying a sailboat together and sailing off to the South Seas when the war ended. I was a good draftsman and was promoted, but I didn't enjoy supervising my fellow workers. Kay and Phyllis had married Turkish architecture students, and were making plans to live in Turkey. Alice had also married. All the boys I knew were going into the service. Everyone was going somewhere! Finally I bought a ticket for Alaska, about the only place one could go during wartime.

Alaska was pristine and beautiful. There were steep mountains, covered with trees down to the water's edge, deep, mysterious fiords and placid little lakes full of trout. In Sitka I got a job in a store and rented a cabin. The cabin wasn't much more than a tarpaper shack, but it was up a lovely green canyon, reached from town by a boardwalk. An oil cook stove burned constantly to keep it warm.

I liked the Alaskan people. They drank a lot, but they were also hard working, adventurous and exuberant. A self-reliant, fun loving bunch, they had tolerant attitudes and uninhibited lifestyles not acceptable in the States until years later. Most Alaskans had come from somewhere else, some giving up traditional careers. An attorney, for instance, had traveled up the Inland Passage in a canoe, with his wife, and set up a business repairing boat motors.

With a vague notion of looking for something more from life than to "settle down and live happily ever after", I had no clear idea what I wanted. For most of my twenty-four years I'd yearned to fall in love, but had almost despaired of finding a man I wanted to marry. Oh, I could be overcome with passionate "love at first sight" upon the appearance of any unattached male between the ages of eighteen and forty, my imagination endowing him with vague, unusual qualities. But after falling out of love just as quickly so many times, I'd about decided I was never going to find whatever I was seeking. (One of my most enduring fantasy heroes was Tarzan. He never talked enough to disillusion me.)

Ike was in the Army and stationed in Sitka. He came into the store where I worked and bought all my favorite records. Then he invited me to the Army post to listen to them. From the moment I met Ike, I somehow never felt an urge to play dumb. Ike had an actual aversion to helpless women. He had been a newspaper reporter before the war, and knew a lot about literature and poetry, things I was trying to understand. We spent hours heatedly discussing ideas, and unorthodox opinions didn't seem to frighten or shock him. Sometimes after hours of debate, Ike would admit he'd agreed with me all along and had only been arguing for fun. My attraction to Ike was more than intellectual though, and while still unable to define whatever I had been looking for in a husband, I knew I'd found it. We were married after knowing each other only a few months.

In those days brides obeyed their husbands. Ike was nine years older than I, and I'd promised to "love and obey" in the marriage ceremony. (Agnostics were accustomed to repeating meaningless words, and it wouldn't have occurred to us to request a change in the ceremony.) However, the first time I asked Ike's permission to do something, he laughed.

"Don't ask me what you can and can't do," he told me. "I'm your husband, not your father." Thus I became a liberated woman before feminism was fashionable.

Soon after we were married, we bought a thirty-foot boat some departing soldiers had put together in their spare time, and began commercial halibut fishing. Our engine was an old truck motor "found" somewhere on the Army post. Salt water corroded the cooling system, causing sudden streams of water to shoot into the air. A supply of corks stopped up such holes, making our engine look like it had warts. Our knowledge of boats was dangerously limited, but being young and fearless, we laughed about harrowing experiences. Luck saved us from piling up on the rocks or being swept out to sea. Financially, the fishing venture was a failure. We would tie up at the dock next to big fishing boats unloading tons of halibut, and place our few little fish on the huge scales. Fish liver, used to make fish liver oil, was sold separately. The weight of our livers was imperceptible on the big scales, but the workers on the dock would laugh and give us a few cents for them. We didn't make enough money to pay for fuel and fishing gear, but both Ike and I loved the experience. Ike remained stationed in Sitka until the war ended.

In 1946, Ike was discharged from the Army in New York. We spent the following summer with his grandmother, who lived deep in the pinewoods on the Eastern Shore of Maryland. Grandmother's place lacked plumbing, electricity, telephones or paved roads. The lethargic little community of Snow Hill, where the population had grown by two in the past 150 years, was about ten miles away. A trip to town with a mule and wagon took an entire day. Time had no meaning that long-ago summer in the pinewoods with Ike's grandmother and her retarded son, Rutledge.

Seances had been a tradition in Ike's family. Grandmother hadn't participated in one for many years, but she agreed to help us communicate with Ike's deceased grandfather, Doctor Vandegrift. When Rutledge had been young the table sometimes became violent if he were in the house. Once it flew up and stuck to the ceiling. Another time it gave Ike's sister a black eye. After that, Rutledge was banished from the house during seances. On this occasion Grandmother sent him down the dirt road to the next farm to spend the evening.

Ike and I sat down to a small table with Grandmother, a frail little lady of eighty-two. Grandfather had built the house himself, apparently forgetting to leave room for stairs, which were a steep, spiral affair inserted in a corner of the parlor. The tiny parlor was crowded with overstuffed furniture, bric-a-brac and faded pictures. The kerosene lamp was dimmed, but I could see our three pair of hands lying on the little table. Except for the sound of the insects of a warm summer evening, the silence was profound in that clearing in the pinewoods.

I didn't believe in seances, and neither Ike nor I believed in ghosts. Nevertheless ghost stories could fill me with an irrational feeling of fear, and I could be reduced to a state of terror by scary movies. I hoped I wouldn't giggle, as I sometimes did when nervous. We sat for a while, and Grandmother began to scold Grandfather affectionately,

"Now, George, the children have come a long way to talk to you. You must say a few words to them."

Finally the table rose up on two legs.

"Is that you, George?" Grandmother asked.

The table came down with a thump, meaning no.

"Is that you, Mary?"

"No," the table again responded.

"Are you anyone we know?"

"No."

"It's nice of you to appear," Grandmother said, "but please go away and let us talk to someone we know."

Finally the table again rose up on two legs and responded with two thumps when asked if we were in communication with Grandfather. Grandmother related news of the family and asked a few questions requiring yes or no answers, none of which seemed significant enough that I remember them. We asked Grandfather's opinion about our plans for the future, but he declined to answer. Finally Grandmother asked if Grandfather had any message.

Two thumps indicated yes.

At last I was about to hear a message from this esteemed doctor who had become a legend in my husband's family.

The table went up on two legs, and Grandmother began, "A, B, C..."

The table came down. On the next repeat of the alphabet it didn't come down until U. Finally the message was spelled out:

"Cut the grass."

I managed not to giggle.

"I realize I haven't kept up the place the way I should lately," Grandmother said. "If I'm still alive next spring I'll plant petunias in the flower bed on the front lawn. Do you have another message?"

"No," the table responded with a final thump. Grandmother seemed to find the seance exhausting, and we didn't ask her to do it again. However we participated in several with Ike's sister and her husband. The table apparently took something from the personality of the participants, for Ike's sister had a flair for the dramatic and would go into a trance during seances. We usually found ourselves talking to dead pirates and notorious murderesses. One evening we were all arguing about how to conduct the seance, and the table sent the message, "Stop bickering." Ike and I later tried to get a table to move by ourselves, but were unsuccessful.

I had no idea what could have moved that table, but even though I believed in science, I did regard nature as infinite and could tolerate paradox and unexplainable phenomena. Nevertheless, I saw no way to fit seances into my view of reality at that time and pushed those episodes off into a remote compartment of my mind. If I occasionally told about them, I did so jokingly, and not expecting to be believed.

*   *   *

Rather than return to his pre-war, newspaper job, Ike wanted to earn a living writing true-detective stories. In those days several magazines were devoted to such accounts. The undertaking was an alternative to the "settling down and living happily ever after" to which I'd felt an aversion. I would help gather information from police records and newspapers, and Ike would write the stories as we traveled through the South. With Ike's mustering-out pay we acquired a pre-war, sixteen-cylinder Lincoln Continental, with a cracked block, and a little old eighteen-foot, canvas-covered house trailer. Our crippled Lincoln had trouble with steep hills, and we made lengthy detours to avoid them. Retreads, at fifty cents apiece, replaced our frequent flat tires. Our trailer had no water hookup, and we carried water in a bucket. Living was somewhat primitive, but the adventure of our undertaking delighted us. We visited small towns and county seats, interviewing sheriffs and constables. Most, flattered by the prospect of their stories appearing in a magazine, eagerly gave details of murder cases they had solved. We once met a sheriff with an apparent "skeleton" in his past, a skeleton that he wanted to keep hidden. When we explained what we were looking for, he angrily ordered us to leave "his county" before dark. Southern sheriffs could exert such authority in those days, and we left cheerfully. Sometimes Southerners were suspicious of us because we were Yankees. When they saw our car and trailer they usually became more friendly, probably deciding we at least weren't a couple of those "Rich-Yankees" who made the trek to Florida each winter.

We met a lot of moonshiners. Murder seemed to be an occupational hazard in that business. By searching through musty old newspaper files, we found murders committed in the last century. Ike wrote accounts of the "dastardly deeds" colorfully described in those old small-town publications. When we happened across a current case, we attended the trial to gather firsthand information. One day we were crossing a railroad track in Elizabeth City, North Carolina. As Ike tried to shift gears, the gearshift came out by the roots, leaving our car and trailer helplessly straddling the tracks. We had arranged for checks from our last stories to be sent to the next town, and had about thirty-seven cents in our pockets.

I hope there's a story in this town," I said with a groan.

"Maybe Grandfather is finally taking an interest in our lives, and is trying to tell us to stop here," Ike offered wryly.

It wasn't the first time we had arrived in a town, broke, and didn't find a check from a magazine waiting at the post office. A job in a restaurant was always easy to get, tiding us over until we sold another story. Ike was soon busy on another story, and a couple of days' tips allowed us to retrieve our Lincoln from the garage where we'd had it towed. After several years traveling through the Southeast, the Lincoln expired, and we settled in Atlanta. Leaving the true-detective stories to Ike, who began using public transportation, I went to work for an architect.

*   *   *

While living in the South, the irrationality of segregation exasperated me In 1948 Henry Wallace ran for President on a platform that included opposition to segregation, and I volunteered my services to the Progressive Party. My politics were liberal in those days. Most liberals were convinced that if socialism were properly administered, and competition were eliminated, the world would be filled with love, kindness and harmony. I remember one of our favorite issues was "slum clearance". We were convinced that if poor people were put in nice houses, they would suddenly become middle class citizens. Campaigning alone in Colored neighborhoods was not considered dangerous in 1948, and I'm sure many Negroes would have felt offended if someone called them black. I once asked a young Negro man to sign my petition to have the Progressive Party placed on the Georgia ballot, and he refused with a look of hatred such as I hadn't encountered in my young life. Maybe he considered my efforts patronizing. I didn't know how to assure him I wasn't opposing segregation for his sake; I was doing it for myself.

Some of the young New York radicals in the Progressive Party were arrogantly patronizing. Unselfishly devoting themselves to liberal causes, they never entertained the slightest doubt about issues they advocated. How could such self-sacrificing idealists be wrong? Opponents could only be motivated by meanness. No one would have uttered the pejorative *nigger*, but Southerners who disagreed with liberal beliefs were called *rednecks* and *bigots*. Raised among unsophisticated people, I understood Southern resentments. Most Southerners of both races were polite to me, even when disagreeing, and signed my petitions to have the Progressive Party slate placed on the Georgia ballot.

One day as I stood on the steps of the Atlanta library collecting signatures, a man stopped and said,

"I'd like to discuss your politics. How about a beer?"

He appeared sincere; I couldn't detect any man-woman type of personal interest in his words or manner.

Reasonable discussion was my favorite pastime.

"O.K.," I agreed, and we went across the street to the Elks Club. I seated myself in a booth, and the man excused himself. A waiter brought me a beer, but the man never returned. He disappeared without a word of political discussion. I sat a while, and after finishing my beer, gathered up my petitions. Collecting signatures as I went, I made my way back to party headquarters.

"How did you escape?" everyone gathered around me to ask, as I walked in the door.

"Escape what?"

They explained while I was in the Elks Club, all the other party workers had been rounded up, taken to jail, mugged and fingerprinted. Full of righteous indignation, they seemed excited by their arrest, rather than frightened. When I went back to the trailer and told Ike, he laughed and promised to bring me a cake with a hacksaw in it if I ended up behind bars. Unlike the others, I felt shaken, and not sure I wanted to go to jail for the Progressive Party. Hearing my views dogmatically expounded by young radicals had dampened my political ardor, and I withdrew from politics.

I've often wondered about that man who bought me a beer. Was he an FBI agent who felt such a polite, friendly girl didn't deserve a police record? Maybe he was an undercover policeman who knew Ike.

*   *   *

Babies had never interested me. When Ike and I married, I was unaware that I wanted children. Nevertheless, during our carefree existence of the past few years, some feminine instinct or hormone had caused me to be overcome with unexpected yearning for a child. Ike had been writing true-detective stories for four years. The income provided a meager existence but was not adequate to support a family. The Korean War started, and Ike had an opportunity to return to active duty in the Army. I urged him to accept. Ike did not feel my desire for children, but we loved each other very much. For me, he returned to the Army. Assigned to public relations, his writing skills were useful. Our son was born a year later, and Ike was surprised to find himself an adoring father. We received orders for Germany, where our second child was born. At that time in Europe new mothers remained flat on their backs in bed for two weeks. After I arrived home from the hospital carrying my two-day-old daughter, I heard my maid brag to her friends,

"Sie gebart Kinder wie eine Katze. Genau wie eine Katze!" (She has babies like a cat. Just like a cat!) The phrase might not sound so wonderful in English, but I could tell from their admiring glances what a flattering thing it was to say in German.

Every moment of the three years we were stationed in Frankfurt was an adventure. I learned German and took up bridge. At German bridge tournaments, we found opportunities to meet Europeans other than the maid and the garbage man. The Army topped off our European adventure by sending us home, first class, on one of the last great passenger liners, the luxurious *SS United States*.

*   *   *

Ike had a drinking problem when we met in Alaska. During his youth he was enthralled by the tough, hard-drinking-reporter legend, admiring Hemingway and Dashiell Hammett and chuckled indulgently over their swashbuckling, alcoholic life styles. Speakeasies and illicit booze had been considered glamorous and exiting. Disdain for anyone who couldn't drink was probably Ike's only macho attitude. Alcohol hadn't been a problem while we were writing true-detective stories, but it was something with which Ike struggled for most of his life. The Army, with a social life based upon cocktail parties and officers' clubs, was an unfortunate choice. By the exercise of will power, Ike always managed to keep his drinking under control—except for periods when he was away from me. I think he depended upon me. When his drinking became excessive, I became emotional and threatened to leave. We both knew it was an empty threat. Certainly, Ike's drinking caused us unhappiness. I hated his stupidity at those times, and felt shame anyone should see him. But Ike only drank sporadically, and most of the time was articulate, considerate and deep-thinking, the only man I ever wanted to marry. We didn't fight or nurse resentments, and although Dr. Dingle might be hard to convince, I knew Ike's drinking had had minimal effect upon the older children, and none upon Tony. I was aware psychiatry attached great significance to guilt. I'd made mistakes during my life, and I regretted them. For instance I should have known I wanted children when I married. I felt bad about urging Ike to go back into the Army. During the McCarthy era, whenever Ike applied for a security clearance I regretted my involvement in radical politics. (An unnecessary regret, because —thanks to that mysterious man who bought me a beer—Ike always got a security clearance.) However, I feared I probably wasn't plagued by the kind of guilt with which psychologists were accustomed to dealing, and I worried that my regrets might not be painful enough to satisfy Dr. Dingle.

I remembered wanting an abortion when I was pregnant with Tony, and the moment in the middle of the night when I thought of putting

Tony in an institution. Those thoughts were fleeting, and I didn't feel guilty about them. However the psychologists would surely consider such lack of guilt abnormal. In fact, they might consider other of my emotional reactions abnormally untypical.

For instance, Ike was sent to Germany six months before I was allowed to join him. A few weeks after I arrived, Ike confessed he'd had an affair. He said the woman was trying to cause trouble and was threatening to tell me. I was annoyed at Ike for his little escapade but I never doubted he loved me. (After World War II, many German girls were eager to find American husbands, a situation many American soldiers thoroughly enjoyed.)

"Bring her here and let her *tell* me," I suggested.

Although skeptical of such a confrontation, Ike went and got her. A nice looking young woman, she stood just inside the door regarding me suspiciously. Ike stood by uneasily. Not sure myself how to proceed, I asked her to sit down.

"Your husband and I have been having an affair," she said.

He told me," I said. "What he did was irresponsible and inconsiderate."

"I told her I was married," Ike said helplessly.

"I'm in love with your husband," she said.

I sat down on the couch, a little stunned, and feeling sorry for her. "I'm so sorry," I said. Had Ike thought telling her he was married excused everything? I would have thought he was too sensitive and considerate to hurt anyone like this. "He would never leave his family. But he shouldn't have… It wasn't right…"

As I struggled to think of something to say, she burst into tears, and turned and ran out of the apartment. (Within six months she married an American Army officer, one who didn't already have a wife.) I'd never told anyone of the incident because of an uneasy feeling about my reaction. I suspected I probably should have pretended some moderate amount of "normal" jealousy.

I had not come into this world a blob of nothing, waiting for environment to shape my character and personality. I knew that by studying garden peas and fruit flies, science had determined we are the result of our genes. (Actually, one might wonder what science knows about the character and personality of garden peas and fruit flies.) Wherever my differences came from, I knew I had been born with them. My nature and personality might not be "average", and I wouldn't enjoy trying to defend them to Dr. Dingle. However most people who knew me seemed to agree I was an unlikely candidate for the couch. Surely I could quickly convince Dr. Dingle I was not emotionally damaged, and that I didn't need any psychiatric treatment. Perhaps the psychologist would then discuss this mysterious medical condition doctors seemed to recognize in Tony. Group therapy seemed as good a place as any to demonstrate my emotional stability.

CHAPTER 7

Do "therapists" try to impose their thinking upon the patient?

I attended that first therapy meeting feeling curious, but not particularly apprehensive. Since I was present "only to allow Tony to form a relationship with someone outside the family", as Dr. Dingle had promised, I planned to be an observer—not a participant. The group consisted of five women, with Dr. Dingle as the moderator. The psychologist said we could talk about anything we wished, or we could sit in silence if we chose. (We would soon discover that sitting silently in the presence of a psychologist is highly uncomfortable —almost an impossibility.) Dr. Dingle suggested we start by each explaining why we had joined the group. I couldn't resist saying,

"My problem is I'm not yet aware I have a problem." Surely the psychologist would realize how ridiculous his statement sounded when hearing it repeated.

One woman was the mother of a child with cerebral palsy and wanted a scientific evaluation of his capabilities, not wishing to expect more of him than he could achieve. The others seemed unhappy. They had complaints— not only about their children—but also about their husbands, their mothers-in-law, San Francisco weather and Army life. I didn't usually choose such unhappy people as friends, and couldn't imagine what anyone might do to alleviate their misery. If Dr. Dingle was willing to try, I had to applaud his effort. Their children seemed normal enough, but didn't behave as their mothers wished. A couple of women complained about nine year old boys who didn't like baths. With a nine-year-old boy of my own at home, I might have been more inclined to drag Guy to a psychologist if he suddenly decided he liked baths. Although I wished Tony would grow up more quickly, I had no intention of sitting around grumbling about him. I did tell a few anecdotes about my children in an attempt to cheer up everyone a little.

For instance, my children liked to sell Kool-Aid with the neighbor children for a penny a glass. We parents supplied the Kool-Aid and then paid the pennies to drink the stuff, all in the interest of training our young entrepreneurs. When Guy was about five, he remarked one evening at dinner.

"Gee, Mommy, Jimmy dropped my lizard in the Kool-Aid today." Then he added, "But I got him out and he was O.K."

Apparently the Kool-Aid was O.K. too. We drank it.

When I told this story in group therapy, a couple of women who seemed unusually concerned about germs shuddered instead of laughing. I also told about Sherry, my feminine little six year old, preoccupied with fairy tales, who complained,

"All the ladies in my story books marry a prince when they grow up, Mommy. But I don't know any princes. Not even one! Are they all used up?"

Sympathizing with a six year old's fondness for fairy tales and fantasies about a prince, I suggested,

"There are still a few around. Prince Charles of England might be the right age for you."

She wanted to know all about him, as she happily made plans to marry the Prince of Wales. She worried whether, as the Queen of England, she should wear her crown while cleaning the castle. She wondered if she should also plan a career; maybe do a little ironing to earn extra money, like Mommy did. Sherry's brother became interested in her plans and asked if she would name her firstborn Guy. The idea of a King Guy the First appealed to him.

"You don't get to name them yourself, silly," she said. "They come with little bracelets on their arms with the names already on them."

This story was more successful with the ladies in group therapy than the one about the lizard in the Kool-Aid. Other than such anecdotes, I had little to say. I had never been good at small talk, but was confident I said enough to demonstrate to the psychologist I didn't have the kind of problems the other women had. While I was in therapy each week, Tony and Dr. Lavalle were in the playroom. Dr. Lavalle wasn't much more talkative than Tony, and Ike and I often wondered what they did together. The first day Dr. Lavalle left the playroom door unlocked, and Tony escaped. I came out to find him making an agile getaway. The psychologist was racing down the hall trying to catch him. Nevertheless, after getting used to the clinic, Tony seemed to look forward to his time there.

Tony had amazed us by announcing, "I talk. One, two, free, four, five. I talk." We were waiting for him to do so. One night he was crying in bed, and I went in to comfort him.

"All-the-way-home hurts," he sobbed.

Looking under his little toe, I found a cut under "the little piggy that went wee-wee-wee all the way home". Tony never allowed us to comfort him in ways we had consoled our other children. He was scornful of kisses as treatment for his hurts, and preferred to rub catsup or mustard on them. After he began talking more, he sometimes spoke of "pictures on the wall" at night, so I know he had an occasional bad dream. Once, he came to get me in the middle of the night and led me into his bed-room. He indicated he wanted me to sit on the floor by his crib and hold his hand until he went back to sleep. He didn't want any nonsense such as kissing.

Tony was growing, but his differences from other children were becoming increasingly apparent. Except for infrequent, startling state-ments, Tony didn't talk. He sometimes went a week without uttering a word. He was good-looking and of average size, but his appearance was immature, and at the age of four he drooled like an infant. Some of his behavior did appear strange

For example, he put his lips to, and tasted metal doorknobs. (I tried it myself and discovered they do have a distinctive taste.) He became fas-cinated by the sound of his own voice, making repeated, meaningless noises, such as "geeee-haw!", in a deep singsong tone. For a time he refused to walk around chairs. Our journey across a crowded waiting room could be tedious, as Tony insisted upon crawling under all the chairs on the way, emerging between the legs of startled people sitting in some of them. Many mischievous children are appealing little hams, their mischief designed Attract attention. Tony's games were obviously for his own amusement.

Like the term modest on the psychological tests, self-esteem seems difficult to define or measure. I've known retarded people with obvious high self-esteem, and attractive, talented people without it. (Psychopaths must have a monumental amount.) Maybe self-esteem is an inherent quality, which an individual can turn into either an asset or a defect. At a very young age, I remember feeling capable of making my own decisions. I often felt awkward in social situations, but as demon-strated by my susceptibility to "genius psychoses", I never lacked self-esteem. Nor did Tony. His self-confidence was apparent to everyone. Some people smiled at his air of boyish independence, but he didn't pay much attention to people and he didn't make friends. I appreciated Dr. Lavalle's companionship for him.

One afternoon Tony found a bucket of paint and painted the washing machine, a neighbor's porch and our dining room floor. When Tony saw our horrified reaction, he ran and got a mop and tried to clean up the mess on the floor. He appeared to realize he'd done something wrong, the first evidence he might be capable of experiencing guilt. That did seem like progress.

Tony hadn't had a temper tantrum for a while. One day shortly before I started group therapy, Tony and I were delivering the ironing I did to help out the family finances, and I didn't turn at the corner where he thought I should. He furiously threw himself over into the back seat, and lit headfirst in a cardboard carton of ironing. I was in heavy traffic and couldn't stop for a few moments. Meanwhile my little tornado, upside down with his head in the ironing, was howling and frantically kicking his feet in the air. When I finally stopped the car and pulled Tony out of the box, he seemed chastened. I hoped landing headfirst in that carton had taught Tony a lesson, and he was learning to control his temper.

*   *   *

One day, Dr. Dingle announced to the group, "We've all sat and complained for three months now. It's time we accomplish something more constructive."

We watched with interest as he strode to the blackboard, a stern expression on his boyish face, picked up a piece of chalk and drew a circle.

"This represents most of our children," he stated. "This represents most of us, constantly exerting control over them." He drew a slightly smaller circle inside the first, and then turned to see if we were following his scientific presentation. "They rebel and break out!" With a flourish, he erased parts of the larger circle, and regarded the group gravely.

"And this," he said, turning back to the blackboard and carefully drawing a big circle, "represents another of our children. We assert no control over this child." The psychologist drew a tiny circle in the middle. "He is frightened and angry." While avoiding looking at any of us, Dr. Dingle printed my name under these last circles.

I stiffened with shock. The psychologist continued writing, adding the words *frightened and angry*.

I stared at the blackboard. *The psychologist believed my treatment of Tony had caused him to become abnormal!* During my forty-one years, people had liked me. Why shouldn't they? Oh, there was the young Negro man in Atlanta who refused to sign my petition. However, his look of hatred hadn't hurt. It was directed at something I represented, not me. But Dr. Dingle didn't even appear to feel any animosity toward me. Being a wife and mother was the role I'd chosen in life. I could have been a good enough architect, but that had been an unimportant, temporary occupation. I chose to be a mother. Now, after knowing me for three months, Dr. Dingle was calmly and impersonally declaring me to be such an inadequate mother that I had warped my little boy's emotional growth. Those circles on the blackboard were apparently intended to add scientific validity to such an awful belief. I felt almost physically ill to think anyone held such a dreadful opinion of me. The other women were watching me solemnly. I sat in stunned silence, barely aware of whatever happened during the rest of the hour.

"We won't meet again until after New Year," I heard the psychologists say as he dismissed us.

I got up and took Tony home in a daze of emotions—anger, hurt, resentment and disbelief—and spent a miserable Christmas holiday. Group therapy, when it resumed after the first of the year, became a dreaded weekly ordeal. Dr. Dingle often mentioned we were all too emotionally involved with our children—except one of us wasn't emotionally involved at all. His accusation of no emotional involvement sounded more malignant than the too much emotional involvement with which the other women were being charged. I refused to give him the satisfaction of arguing over the ridiculous allegation. Such argument would accomplish nothing. How I could prove to anyone that I loved my children. Other than an occasional question or comment to the other women, I sat each week and grimly endured the hour.

One day I reported Tony didn't seem to have tantrums anymore. A look of annoyance passed across Dr. Dingle's face. Why should he be disappointed for Tony to stop having tantrums? Was he trying to prove some theory? Did he not want Tony to improve, except in response to some psychiatric treatment? I remembered the silly "cures" of highly intelligent, "withdrawn" children described in old psychology books. When Tony grew up to be such a child, I would feel obligated to protest he was not "cured" by something so absurd as his mother's participation in group therapy.

The group had been meeting for about five months when Dr. Dingle asked all the husbands to come in for an interview. Ike, of course, was willing to do anything that might help Tony. He spoke with the head of the clinic, a Colonel Mann. Afterwards, Ike reported the psychologists were dissatisfied with my behavior. They protested I didn't talk, as the other women did. Surely the psychologists didn't actually approve of all that complaining! I remembered Dr. Dingle had promised in the beginning I was there "only to allow Tony to form a relationship with someone outside the family". The thought of his duplicity galled me.

Ike mentioned to Colonel Mann I'd read every psychology book in the local library.

"She did? She didn't tell us that," said the colonel. "You see! Your wife doesn't tell us anything."

After that Ike went with us to the clinic every week and talked to Colonel Mann. Ike didn't mind. In those days mother was considered responsible for a child's emotional development, and no one was accusing Tony's father of anything. When it came to the subject of my relationship with the children, however, Ike was an unwavering defender.

Sherry came home from school and reported her second-grade teacher had asked the children to write a story about their families. Sherry had written,

"Everyone in my family goes to psychiatrists except me." (Her nine-year-old brother had become fascinated with psychiatry. He read psychology books, and participated in family arguments on the subject. She put him in the same category with the rest of us.)

Sherry's teacher had recently told me that Sherry was still writing some of her letters backwards. Reversals, the teacher had assured me, were merely a sign of immaturity. Nevertheless, Sherry was reversing after the other children had stopped. If she continued much longer, the teacher warned, "Something would have to be done about it". I wondered what could be done, other than allowing her to mature. No one seemed able to do anything about Tony's immaturity, which made Sherry's look insignificant.

One day as I listened to the other women, I realized Ike was the only father still coming to the clinic. These women had complained about their husbands' treatment of their children. I on the other hand, had reported Ike to be the kindest, most patient of fathers. Nevertheless, Ike's continued weekly attendance at the clinic seemed to suggest the psychologists considered us the most dysfunctional family of the group. (Actually, I don't think the term "dysfunctional family" was yet fashionable, but there was no doubt the psychologists felt our family needed fixing.) Colonel Mann had again protested to Ike I was uncommunicative, bringing up the fact that I hadn't even told them I'd read psychology books.

"You don't believe I caused Tony to be abnormal, do you?" I would tearfully ask Ike.

"No, of course not."

"Why won't they tell us what is wrong with Tony? They've said he isn't retarded. They insist he is above average intelligence. What else could be wrong with him?"

"I don't know. Why don't you ask Dr. Dingle? The psychologists complain you don't talk enough."

I had never emerged from any confrontation feeling successful. When emotionally upset, my slow-motion mind prevented me from thinking what I should have said until a week later. The prospect of a confrontation with a glib psychologist left me weak with fear and dread. Nevertheless, I finally went to group therapy one day determined to speak.

"Do you have evidence children like Tony don't grow up to be normal," I demanded," or do you object to him merely because he isn't average?"

Dr. Dingle and the other women looked startled.

"What's wrong with Tony?" I persisted. "Is he mentally retarded?"

"No, he's very bright - extremely bright!" While skeptical of other things psychologists said, for some reason I always believed them when they declared Tony to be extremely bright.

"How do you know? Did you give him an IQ test?"

"Tony isn't testable right now, but we can tell by looking he is very alert."

"Do you suspect Tony of being psychotic?"

"Of course not!"

"Then what is wrong with him?"

"He's emotionally retarded."

I had never heard of the term.

"My other son was like Tony until he was three. Was he emotionally retarded?" I asked—unable to keep sarcasm out of my voice

"*I* think so."

"Oh for heaven's sake," I exclaimed. Then I took a deep breath and forced myself to attempt a less contentious tone.

"Tony hasn't developed much interest in people yet. It's a quality everyone has to differing degrees. Couldn't Tony have been born that way?"

I was confident people created by scientists would be a disaster. Psychologists didn't seem to share my confidence in nature, regarding scientifically trained specialists to be the proper judges of what people should and should not be. Children's personalities were considered blank pages at birth. Most psychologists were convinced that—with correct parenting as defined by twentieth-century professionals—everyone could be molded into similar, successful, untroubled, perennially contented useful citizens.

"No," Dr. Dingle stated, "children are not born that way."

"You believe I did something to Tony?"

"I believe it was something you didn't do."

He was obviously referring to his repeated charge that I was not emotionally involved with my children.

"Sometimes I feel terrified about Tony. *I know* I didn't cause his slow development," I said. "If there is something wrong, it's physical. The medical profession should stop wasting time like this, and try to find out what it is."

Dr. Dingle looked uncomfortable.

"People with emotional problems are unhappy," I argued. I turned to the other women, who had been sitting in silence, listening to my confrontation with the psychologist. "You are all aware of your unhappiness aren't you?" I asked.

They agreed.

"Well I've always had more fun than most people."

"That seems important to you," the psychologist suggested cunningly.

"Oh, for crying out loud!" He seemed determined to make something sinister out of my every remark. Then I added in exasperation, "I don't understand how you psychologists can believe some little event in a child's life could actually prevent him from growing up normally."

"What do you mean by some little event?" Dr. Dingle asked.

I glared at him, unwilling to suggest any.

"Why do you suppose Tony does things like lie down on the floor at Sunday School?" he persisted.

"I suppose Sunday School bored him!"

I realized nothing I might say would make any difference to this psychologist. He had become committed to some theory before ever seeing Tony or me. But surely I was entitled to know my child's diagnosis!

"Have you never seen another child like Tony?" I asked.

Dr. Dingle shook his head uneasily.

I didn't believe him. Other doctors had seemed to suspect some diagnosis. They seemed interested in a child who might have an unusual reaction to a fountain pen spinning on the floor like a top; a child who took things apart and whose antecedents went to college, got good grades, and professed some unusual attitude toward religion; a child who ignored other children; a child who made symmetrical designs with blocks.

"When I first spoke to Dr. Berger, he didn't think there was necessarily anything wrong with Tony," I said.

"Just what did Dr. Berger tell you?" Dr. Dingle demanded, rising from his chair.

Maybe the two psychologists disagreed about Tony. If so, I felt loyalty and gratitude toward Dr. Berger, who hadn't seemed devious.

"Nothing," I mumbled, lowering my eyes. Dr. Berger hadn't actually told me anything. And if he had inadvertently revealed optimism by his tone of voice, I wouldn't tell on him.

The psychologist strode across the room and stood menacingly over me.

"You know," he warned, "Tony is not going to grow up—or talk—until you do something."

I knew what he meant by "do something". Psychology books described how feelings of hostility, and incestuous thoughts about one's parents dominate most people's lives. Dr. Dingle was apparently furious because I refused to confess any such feelings. Freud was the discoverer of denial. Patients who refused to admit to one of his imaginative diagnoses were accused of denial, a convenient concept for therapists. Faced with an accusation of being in denial, who could win an argument with an analyst?

I sat silently, intimidated by Dr. Dingle's anger. The other women, who had momentarily found my encounter with the psychologist more interesting than their own problems, waited a few minutes and then resumed their usual complaints.

CHAPTER 8

Who is abusing whom?

Ike tried to discuss with Colonel Mann what Dr. Dingle had said to me.

"Your wife was mistaken," the colonel told Ike. "Dr. Dingle would never have said such things. And I can assure you he wouldn't get angry," How could he be so certain Dr. Dingle never became angry? Did he consider psychologists immune to such emotions?

It had been a year since I first took Tony to the pediatrician. Tony's unexpected behavior had always seemed funny to us. One reason was probably Tony's attitude. Our other two children became offended and cried if we laughed at them too much, but Tony seemed to enjoy it. Full of fun himself, Tony loved to tease. He would sometimes hide in the bushes when I called him from the yard. When I found him, he would laugh with delight at his cleverness. During the time I was attending group therapy I still tried to find humor in Tony's mischief, but I was often on the verge of tears. He continued to break the glass out of the door when he couldn't get it open. Ike had replaced it several times. We tried to discipline Tony, but were unable to find effective punishments. We had to be careful not to punish him to relieve our fear and frustration or to satisfy people who considered him spoiled. It's understandable how the myth about child abuse causing retardation originated. Children who do not respond to normal discipline are frustrating. I'm sure some have been abused.

My mother had knit Tony a pillow, which looked like a big bug. Tony, nearly five, was still in diapers. He would run and get his pillow, and lie on the floor with it under his head while I changed his diapers.

"Will you expect me to change your diapers after you start riding your first motorcycle, you rascal?" I sometimes exclaimed.

Tony, his head on his pillow, would smile impishly at my frustration. He also slept with his pillow.

"Find piddow," Tony said one night at bedtime.

I searched the house. Tony followed me repeating, "find piddow" more insistently.

"Everyone help find Tony's pillow," I urged, and we began looking in the yard. It was getting dark and we couldn't find a flashlight. (Flashlights were one of the things Tony kept dismantled.) By this time Tony was in tears and screaming,

"Find piddow! Find piddow!"

"Maybe we can use candles," I suggested. "If that pillow comforts Tony at night, we must find it." Insecure was not a term I would have ascribed to Tony. Nevertheless it was one of child psychology's favorite themes. I was determined to do everything possible to avoid any accusation of causing Tony to be insecure.

Keeping candles lit while walking around the yard was difficult. We improvised cardboard windbreaks and searched for more than an hour. Tony began to enjoy the hunt and stopped crying. Although we didn't find the pillow, he finally went to bed without it. We found it the next morning, in plain sight, up in a tree.

The next evening at bedtime Tony asked for his pillow. I took it from a closet where I'd kept it safely hidden all day.

"No!" he objected as he grabbed it from me and ran and threw it out the window. "Find piddow," he repeated.

"No, Tony, no candles tonight," I told him. "Go out and get your pillow if you want to sleep with it."

Tony went to bed without his pillow and seemed indifferent about sleeping with it after that.

*   *   *

Tony used to stop up the toilet by flushing down his blocks. We'd call the *rotorooter* man to dislodge them. One evening we were in the bathroom watching the *rotorooter* machine, and heard a noise in the living room. Rushing out, we found Tony with a hack saw from the *rotorooter* man's toolbox, enthusiastically sawing a leg off a table. In that moment of confusion the *rotorooter* man decided he couldn't do the job this time. We'd have to call a plumber. He said he wouldn't charge for his unsuccessful efforts. "If you don't want money, we might give you Tony," we joked.

Tony was so cute and bright looking no one could resist laughing, and the *rotorooter* man laughed too. He retreated in mock alarm, saying,

"The only people who might have use for that young man would be some demolition company."

*   *   *

Tony was rarely sick. His few childhood illnesses were so mild as to be almost unnoticeable. However, he got a bad cold that spring, and I took him to the pediatric clinic. While we were waiting, he investigated the scales by the reception desk. After a couple of minutes, he came and handed me a piece of it. I tried to replace it on the scales, but couldn't find where it fit. I gave it to the nurse and apologized. (During Tony's childhood I spent much of my time apologizing for him.) She tried to replace it, but decided a screw must be missing. Surely Tony hadn't been near the scales long enough to unscrew anything! Sometimes though, mechanical devices seemed to disintegrate spontaneously whenever

Tony approached. We went in to see the doctor. When she tried to look down Tony's throat, he bit the tongue depressor in two and kicked the doctor in the face.

"He shouldn't act like this at his age," she exclaimed.

"We go to psychologists every week," I said.

"That's good," she said, and continued to examine Tony while keeping out of range of his feet. "How do you like the Child Guidance Clinic?"

"I hate it."

"You should be grateful for such help."

"I can force myself to go; I can't make myself like it," I protested.

Then I exclaimed in exasperation, "I always thought one should be frank and open when dealing with psychiatry. But that psychologist goes into a big old purple funk whenever I try to start a candid discussion. He acts like he'd rather hide under his desk!"

The doctor laughed. It was refreshing to see a doctor laugh. There wasn't much gaiety around the psychiatric clinic. Everyone, doctors and patients, were grimly taking themselves and their emotions so very seriously.

"They've said Tony is extremely bright and he isn't psychotic," I said. "Do you know of anything else that be wrong with him?

"Well, childhood schizophrenia."

"But they said he isn't psychotic."

"The psychiatrists would know more about that than I would," she said, turning her attention back to Tony. The doctor treated Tony's cold without further comment. As we went out through the waiting room, several people were on their hands and knees around the scales, presumably still searching for that missing screw. I'd already done all the apologizing I could stomach for one day, and I took Tony's hand and hurried out the door with him.

*   *   *

Food was an important item in Tony's life, and cookies were near the top of his list. He could enter any kitchen and spot the cookie jar, regardless of its disguise. He silently and unobtrusively darted up and snatched cookies from strangers in public places, leaving them staring at their empty hands, wondering where their cookie went. Cookie snatching may have been what he had in mind the day he got into more serious trouble. For me it was a last straw. On this particular afternoon I couldn't find Tony in the yard. I ran up the hill behind the house calling him, and met a man leading him down the road by the hand. Tony was crying. The man declared indignantly,

"He scared me to death! I thought he was a burglar. He walked right into my house. I had a gun. I almost shot him!"

I apologized and took Tony home. In a few minutes a policeman knocked on the door.

"Do you have a boy named Anthony here?" he asked. I nodded. "An escapee from juvenile hall?" he continued.

Tony, traces of tears still on his dusty little cheeks, stamped his foot and made threatening motions at the policeman.

"Get out a here," Tony warned, advancing menacingly. He stopped just out of the policeman's reach and stamped his little foot again. "You get out a here!"

"He's only four years old! How could he have escaped from Juvenile hall?" I asked.

The policeman stood in the door without answering, a look of disapproval on his face, watching Tony's efforts to drive him away. I doubted he was really searching for an escapee from juvenile Hall. Surely four-year-olds would be incapable of such breakouts. Perhaps the man who brought Tony home had called the police before discovering how small his "burglar" was. Maybe the policeman was trying to emphasize that housebreaking was a serious offense, and trying to convince Mother she should do something about her young delinquent, so he wouldn't end up in juvenile hall one day. Psychologists weren't the only ones who felt I should do something about Tony.

"That young man needs a good spanking," the policeman finally said, as he turned and left.

I tried to laugh about the predicaments my four year old could get into, but found myself crying again. What did the psychologists think might happen to Tony? He was a notorious cookie snatcher. Did they think he might grow up to be a criminal, for heaven's sake? Surely somewhere I could find a doctor who would discuss this mysterious thing doctors seemed to think might be wrong with my little boy.

A friend recommended a civilian pediatrician. As I met the new doctor in his office, I tried to explain that the psychologists claimed my little boy was extremely bright and wasn't psychotic. By this time I was unable to talk about Tony without crying.

"What else might be wrong with him when he grows up?" I asked, struggling with tears.

"Well, he might not get married or something like that," the doctor said.

He seemed puzzled at the bitterness with which I spoke of Dr. Dingle.

"If you are undergoing therapy somewhere and are angry at the psychologist, you should tell him," he said. "In therapy feelings of anger must be brought into the open."

The pediatrician didn't feel qualified to discuss Tony's condition and obtained an appointment for me with a well-known child psychiatrist.

I hoped Tony would get married when he grew up. It seemed a silly thing to worry about while he was only four years old. I'd read Freud was the first to suggest mother was responsible for her son's homosexuality. He made his discovery by psychoanalyzing Leonardo da Vinci, who had been dead for some five hundred years and was reportedly homosexual. Leonardo didn't write an autobiography, but he did leave one account of a dream. Dreams were Freud's specialty. There had been

other dream-analyzers, but Freud claimed to be the first to do it scientifically. (Freud was disappointed that he never received a Nobel Prize
for his scientific discoveries.) Leonardo had dreamed a vulture came
and flicked its tail on his lips. Everyone familiar with psychiatric theory
must be aware of Freud's scientific discovery that a bird's tail, as well as
a snake, a cigar and just about any other similarly shaped object, is a
symbol for a penis. In Egyptian hieroglyphics a vulture is the symbol for
mother. Leonardo was Italian, but Freud thought he might know
Egyptian hieroglyphics. (Actually, the Rosetta Stone hadn't been translated, and no one knew Egyptian hieroglyphics in Leonardo's day.)
According to Freud's analysis, Leonardo's dream indicated his mother
had stolen his manhood, thus accounting for Mona Lisa's smug smile.
Someone later discovered Freud had used a faulty translation, from
Italian to German, of Leonardo's dream. The bird in Leonardo's dream
wasn't a vulture, but a kite. In Egyptian hieroglyphics a kite is only a
symbol for that species of bird, nothing else. It was further asserted that
Leonardo, who was illegitimate, spent his infancy and childhood with
his father and stepmother, not his mother. However Freud found a
painting by Leonardo with two Mona Lisa's, both sporting smug smiles.
He continued to insist mothers cause homosexuality. Since Western
society became permeated with psychoanalytic theory early in this century, psychiatry had been busy trying to fix all deviations from average,
including sexual orientation.

I would have found it difficult to worry about Tony's sexual orientation, if that was what the pediatrician was questioning. Even at the age
of four, Tony's every movement and gesture seemed to suggest exaggerated masculinity.

*   *   *

The office of the psychiatrist was located in a building with a spectacular view of San Francisco Bay. *Please, please let this psychiatrist at*

least be candid! How could I trust a doctor who seemed to be keeping something from me? Why was medical profession behaving so deviously? The psychiatrist invited me to leave Tony in the waiting room and come into his office.

Leave Tony in the waiting room? Alone? The psychiatrist didn't seem to have a receptionist. A couple of chairs and a lamp seemed to be the only furniture. Maybe there wasn't much for Tony to destroy or dismantle. "Be a good boy," I admonished with a display of confidence as I put Tony on a chair. He looked angelic. Although alert looking, and curious about everything, there was never a trace of guile on Tony's bright, innocent little face.

A plate-glass wall of the psychiatrist's office overlooked a small-boat harbor. I seated myself in a big comfortable chair. The psychiatrist, a likeable, friendly man, listened as I told about the Child Guidance Clinic and my disagreements with Dr. Dingle.

"Dr. Dingle says Tony is very bright," I explained.

The psychiatrist sat waiting for me to continue.

"Extremely bright!" I said.

The psychiatrist still didn't react. Probably all mothers who consulted him considered their children to be extremely bright. I didn't know how to suggest Tony's superior intelligence apparently had some mysterious relationship to his unusual development. When I tried to talk about some of Tony's mischief, the psychiatrist kept glancing nervously toward his waiting room, where Tony was sitting unattended.

"I honestly don't understand why you consulted me," he finally said.

"I want to know what might happen to Tony."

"I've seen many of these children end up in institutions," he said gravely.

I stared at him in horror, afraid to ask what he meant. I couldn't think of any reason for putting people in institutions other than retardation, psychosis or criminal acts.

"Do you believe children are born like Tony, or do you think their condition is the result of something in their environment?" I finally managed to ask.

"There are psychiatrists who believe children are born like this. I'm not one of them."

That was at least an honest answer. I wondered if he would take offence if I asked where I might find one of those psychiatrists who disagreed with him? It probably wouldn't be very tactful.

"The purpose of psychotherapy is to get to know yourself," the psychiatrist said, apparently still puzzled about what I wanted.

"But I already know myself better than most people do. And it's damned unpleasant having that psychologist sit around waiting to pounce upon one of my so-called problems."

"Therapy is not like a social relationship. If you get angry at the psychologist, don't keep your feelings to yourself. Tell him exactly what you think of him." After a moment's hesitation he added, "What would you like to tell him?"

"I'd like to tell that pompous little fugitive from the *Organization Man* he has more problems than I have!" The recent book, The *Organization Man*, criticized psychological tests among other things. Most psychiatric theories were accepted with religious fervor in those days, but I eagerly read anything I could find critical of psychology.

"What could telling that psychologist off possibly accomplish?" I asked.

The psychiatrist stared at me. Not a muscle of his face moved. He sat staring at me. I was reminded of the time a year ago in the first pediatrician's office. Something about me, my grades in school, had seemed to suggest Tony's strange diagnosis. Other people's thoughts had always been a mystery to me. I've recently read the difference between analytical and intuitive brains lessens as we get older, and linear thinkers sometimes acquire more intuitive abilities. Under the awful trauma of the past year, my mind seemed to have made a quantum leap. To my surprise, I felt insight into this psychiatrist's thinking. I knew he was finally recognizing Tony's mysterious diagnosis.

"Is Tony a rocker?" the psychiatrist suddenly asked. "Or have you ever noticed him attach something to a piece of string and spin it?"

"He rocks his head back and forth before he goes to sleep, but I've never seen him spin anything."

"Did you work before you were married?"

That first pediatrician had wanted to know what type of work I did in Alaska.

"I was an architectural draftsman."

"And your husband?"

"He used to be a newspaper reporter."

The psychiatrist smiled and nodded. He suggested sympathetically,

"You consulted me because you don't believe they have been honest with you at the psychiatric clinic, didn't you?"

"They have refused to tell me anything."

The psychiatrist suggested I try another clinic, Langly Porter Psychiatric Institute. The last thing I wanted was to be treated at another clinic. I was looking for someone to tell me all they knew about this mysterious diagnosis they suspected.

"Would you be willing to take Tony as a patient?" I asked. In spite of his belief that Tony's condition was caused by environment, this psychiatrist did seem sincere and candid.

"Do you think you could afford my fees, several hundred dollars a month?"

"We have some money saved. I would pay anything to learn something definite about Tony."

"Actually, I don't have any free time right now. But if you'll give me the name of your psychologist, I'd like to phone him."

"Please don't do that," I said. "He's already angry at me. He'd probably kick Tony right out of the clinic."

"I don't think you have to worry about that! No, I'm going to phone him," repeated the psychiatrist. He sounded provoked.

Not again! Please God not again! The psychologist's annoyance did seem directed at Dr. Dingle, not me. Nevertheless, this doctor visit was going to be as futile as the others. It was like a nightmare, where one is aware of dreaming, but powerless to stop the terrible events from running their awful course. If only there were something I could say to stop this doctor from dismissing me without discussing Tony!

"I read all the psychology books in the local library," I confessed, just in case the psychiatrist was angry with me for withholding information.

The psychiatrist looked startled.

"Now, I'm not going to charge you full price for your consultation today," he said, ignoring my confession. "Fifteen dollars will be enough."

It had happened again. He expected me to leave.

"I think I've made a wonderful adjustment to life, considering the way I am," I defended myself. "I could have been an alcoholic like my father." Secretly, I still preferred "however I was" to being normal, and that was the truth! In any case, no one could possibly accuse me of withholding information now.

The psychiatrist only looked bewildered.

Reluctantly, and feeling defeated, I got up and collected Tony from the waiting room. For some reason, he hadn't found anything to dismantle. I had apparently hit bargain day, and the psychiatrist had only charged me half- price. However, the only advice he'd given was to go tell Dr. Dingle exactly what I thought of him. But the psychiatrist planned to reveal my feelings over the phone, and Dr. Dingle would probably already be aware of them anyway.

Over the years, I made other attempts to find a doctor who would talk to me. The results were similar. Psychiatrists would not contradict each other, and medical doctors would not interfere with their colleagues, the psychiatrists. The only medical treatment available to Tony seemed to be psychotherapy.

CHAPTER 9

Do traumatic childhoods actually cause damaged adults?

I had spent my life avoiding confrontations. I had never told anyone off. However, this was what both the psychiatrist and the pediatrician had recommended. After brooding about Dr. Dingle for a week, I went to the next therapy session determined to try. The other women seemed to sense something amiss and didn't begin their usual round of complaints. Dr. Dingle, however, had been warned by the psychiatrist and was expecting me. He showed no surprise when I erupted the moment we were seated, instead of sinking into my usual brooding silence.

"You said Tony was the first child you'd heard of like him," I accused him. "That's not true. There are others, aren't there?"

"Yes," he admitted.

"You also said Tony wouldn't grow up until I do something. You had no right to say such a thing. Some authorities disagree," I bluffed. I hoped the psychologist was unaware that I had been unable to locate such a doctor.

"That's true," he again admitted. "It was only my opinion."

"I'm not interested in your psychiatric opinions. They are just a bunch of theories. I want facts. What happens to children like Tony when they grow up?"

"Well, sometimes they don't relate to people properly."

"By properly, I suppose you mean the way you do it?" I asked scornfully. *Did that qualify as telling him off?* My tone was really sarcastic.

I was aware that relating to people was not something at which everyone in my family was talented. Nevertheless, some of those who had to make the greatest effort were fine human beings and led satisfactory lives. Humanity consists of lawyers and poets, physicists and metaphysicians, innovators and conservatives, all adding up to a vibrant but stable society. It seemed to me there was reason for all sorts of people in this world. However, I felt unprepared to defend any family traits to a psychologist.

Dr. Dingle was silent and I continued,

"What do you mean by relate to people properly?"

"Sometimes they have to be institutionalized."

That ominous threat again.

"What did that civilian psychiatrist tell you?" he continued.

This was my effort to tell Dr. Dingle exactly what I thought of him, and I couldn't allow him to gain the initiative. I swallowed my horror at the thought of Tony in an institution and replied boldly,

"Doctors don't have to tell me things. I can read their minds. I can read yours, too," I warned

Dr. Dingle looked uncomfortable, and I dearly wished I could read doctors' minds. I only knew there was something everyone was refusing to discuss.

"You have sometimes intimated one of my so-called problems is I don't trust people, namely you," I continued. "Well I've answered all your questions, whether I considered them any of your business or not. All you've done in return is worry about what some other doctor might tell me." *Did that qualify as telling him off? It had only taken a few minutes.* The psychologist was watching me with an unreadable expression on his face and didn't appear particularly told off. "And in addition to all that, I don't like you very much," I added lamely, unable to think of anything more. I probably hadn't done a very good job, but I was exhausted. I collapsed into silence.

Dr. Dingle still didn't say anything. The other women sat a few minutes before regaining their voices. Then one of them burst out with one of their typical complaints.

"Someone called from school this week to report my daughter had been bitten by a horse," she announced.

More details disclosed her eight-year-old daughter, who loved animals and was afraid of nothing, had run up to pet a policeman's horse. Her hand accidentally bumped into its teeth, and the teachers were concerned the horse might have bitten her. The mother considered being bitten by a horse, right in the middle of a big city like San Francisco, a good example of why her daughter needed psychiatric treatment. I was tempted to suggest that the mother had more problems than the daughter, but would never have said such a thing to anyone. Emotionally drained by my confrontation with the psychologist, I didn't pay much attention for the rest of the meeting.

*   *   *

"If any of you want to discuss your children with me privately, I've set aside Tuesday afternoons for that purpose," Dr. Dingle announced to the group several times during the next few weeks. I wasn't about to accept an invitation to talk to him alone. Colonel Mann had insisted Dr.

Dingle didn't say things I had heard. If Dr. Dingle wanted to declare Tony's development the result of my emotional maltreatment, he'd have to do it with the other women as witnesses. Actually, psychologists terrified me—with their authority to make official pronouncements about a person's mental state. We all form opinions about the people we meet. When one acquires a psychology degree, these personal opinions were apparently elevated to the status of scientific, medical diagnoses. I had read of psychologists describing parents with unhealthy attitudes. They spoke of over-protective parents and rejecting parents. Then, there were those parents who didn't fit either category, the inconsistent parents. I myself hadn't doubted such verdicts if made by a professional. Now I wondered, what gave doctors or psychologists the ability to make such judgments?

Dr. Dingle claimed I wasn't emotionally involved with my children. I could protest that I was, but had no illusions about which of us the world was likely to believe. What if Dr. Dingle decided to pronounce me a raving psychotic? Would anyone pay attention to my protests, words of a mere layman?

Most mental illness is diagnosed by "aberrant thinking", with no detectable physical pathology, and society has granted psychiatrists the authority to define "aberrant thinking". Homosexuality was once considered pathological—until gay activists forced psychiatry to take it off their "mental illness" list. I'm sure many psychiatrists regard some religious beliefs as delusional, but are prudent enough not to label such an overwhelming majority of the population as "mentally ill". These days when I hear of a patient involuntarily confined to a mental institution declare, "I'm not insane; it's the doctors who are crazy," I consider that a real possibility.

As the psychiatrist had predicted, Dr. Dingle did not kick Tony out of the clinic. Once, he did suggest uneasily we might like to quit therapy. Suspicious of any suggestion he might offer, I ignored him. I was frightened for Tony. The fear was there in my stomach like a physical pain every morning. It was there if I awoke in the middle of the night. Any parent who has watched anxiously over a critically ill child might guess how that agonizing uncertainty would feel if prolonged day after day, week after week, month after month, year after year. The psychiatric clinic seemed to offer the only medical treatment available. Frightened as we were, it would have been hard to turn our backs upon medical science. Raised in a family of doctors, Ike would have found it especially difficult. Science was the religion of our time and psychiatry was one of the most revered. I was struggling against another of my unorthodox opinions: the growing conviction that this particular so-called science was mostly nonsense. We continued taking Tony to the clinic. Dr. Dingle abandoned overt attempts to locate my problem, but one day he gazed up at the ceiling, and addressing no one in particular, said,

"It's awful to want to be independent and dependent at the same time!"

Such agony looked inappropriate on Dr. Dingle's round, boyish face. The psychologist probably considered me too independent for a normal female. I remembered the castration complex Freud claimed afflicted little girls. Feminism was not yet respectable in the early 60's, and independent women were sometimes accused of wishing they were men. Certainly, most of the world probably agreed with Dr. Dingle that women shouldn't be too self-reliant. A couple of caustic remarks about the psychologist's painful, ambiguous feelings came to mind. They remained unsaid. I limited my comments to an occasional description of Tony's progress.

One week I became aware that, for various reasons, all the other women would be absent from the next meeting. I'd have to spend the hour alone with Dr. Dingle. A whole hour! I'd probably nervously blurt out some crazy remark—something he could use as evidence of my emotional abnormality. On the dreaded day I showed up, tense with apprehension, but grimly determined not to let the psychologist know I feared him. Dr. Dingle suggested since there were only two of us we skip therapy for that week. He seemed uneasy and avoided my gaze. Could the psychologist be as afraid of me as I was of him? Maybe I'd convinced him I could read his mind. Fancy me possessing the ability to intimidate someone—and of all people, a doctor!

*   *   *

As I read psychiatry books, I'd come to realize most psychiatric patients become convinced they were starved for affection during an unhappy childhood. Dr. Dingle wouldn't have approved of my childhood, but I honestly didn't remember it as unhappy. I was the eldest of four children. Mother was busy doing the work required of mothers in those days. No one worried about how we related to our peer group or whether we were living up to our capabilities. Unaware of the formulas of child psychology, my parents accepted our deviations from average, allowed us to make decisions, and assumed growing up came naturally. We attended school and did our household chores, and would have been amazed to learn adults might try to understand us. We enjoyed the freedom of living in a small town. Pulling our wagon around the hills and pastures, we pretended to be explorers on dangerous journeys. We dammed the creeks and waded in them. My happy childhood memories include the sounds of birds and small animals in the quiet of the woods, wild flowers, and the different smells of spring and summer in the sunny fields. We built a tree house in an oak tree, where we published a newspaper. Leaving our little bundles of paper on the neighbors' steps, we were undiscouraged when our scandalous reports of everyone's mis-deeds disappeared into the trash unread. In winter we entertained our-selves by cutting paper-dolls from catalogues. Copying the crises ridden lives of radio soap-opera characters, we enacted stories with them.

One day when I was about five I remember an urge to examine the contents of a jewelry box Mother kept on her dresser. Mother confined us to her room when we misbehaved, and it occurred to me such punishment might offer opportunity for a leisurely examination of the treasures in that box. I asked for a glass of milk and dropped it on the floor. Mother got a mop and began to clean up the mess.

"Damn milk," I said. I'd never uttered this word before and was sure it would result in punishment.

"Little girls shouldn't swear," Mother scolded absently.

I pulled a stack of pots and pans off a shelf, scattering them over the floor with a loud bang and clatter.

"What has gotten in to you today?" Mother exclaimed. She felt my forehead to see if I was feverish.

I deliberately knocked by sister down, making her cry.

"Go to my room and stay there until you can behave," Mother finally ordered. Suspicious of my quick compliance, she checked after a few minutes and found me sitting on top of the dresser draped with chains, pins, rings and necklaces. She finally lost patience and spanked me.

One day my brother and sister and I were playing store. Our merchandise consisted of cans of acorns on an assortment of boards, stacked on bricks and boxes. Unaccustomed to adults participating in our games, we were surprised when two Indian women in long calico skirts stopped to examine our store. They were accompanied by a couple of children our age that watched us with solemn big brown eyes. The women were talking in their language. We ceased playing, three barefoot, grubby little kids, and stood looking at them.

"How much?" one of the women asked in English.

"Pennies?" suggested my enterprising five-year-old brother. We had been using rocks for money.

They conferred, and then offered us three real copper pennies in exchange for our entire stock of acorns.

"We come back tomorrow," they promised. We spent the rest of the day scampering around the hills gathering buckets of acorns. I don't know if we were the only individuals to be thus exploited by Indians. Their children apparently weren't interested in picking up acorns at that price. However, for several summers we were thrilled to gather them for a penny a bucket.

As we grew older we enjoyed working. We pulled our wagon around town, selling produce from the family vegetable garden. We picked prunes, baby-sat, did chores for the neighbors, sold magazines, worked in the movie theater and in the harvest of local crops. We undoubtedly had less money than most people in town, but we didn't feel poor. We took a can of fruit to church at Christmas for the poor people. If we ever became the recipients of that food collected for the poor people, my parents never told us.

We always had enough to eat. My father liked to hunt and fish, and during the depression we ate illegal fish and game. We all loved family camping trips, and the most exciting were those times we thought the game warden was pursuing us. However I've since learned many people in town were aware of Daddy's poaching. If the game warden had wanted, he surely would have had no trouble catching my parents, with their four children, baby bottles and diapers, two hound dogs, a cat, a canary and our camping gear piled into an old open touring car. We spent time in the car like normal rowdy kids, until we had a flat tire or broke down. Then we got out and sat by the side of the road, silently, and without moving. Daddy's temper was on a short leash when the car wasn't running. Once it was fixed we resumed our noisy bickering and teasing.

I wouldn't want to give the impression we were just a happy, carefree, fun-loving family. Daddy was uncommunicative and must have found it difficult to show emotion. I have no clear picture of him as a person, what he felt, wished for or believed. His drinking seemed to be a part of my earliest memories. We would awaken in the middle of the night to hear Mother and Daddy quarreling. Sometimes Mother would get us out of bed, and all of us except Daddy would go stay with friends. Neither my parents nor their friends were sophisticated enough to be aware such experiences might damage a child's psyche. They wouldn't have known the meaning of the word psyche. We were pretty much ignored at those times. The truth is, children are adaptable, and we learned to cope. We accepted disruptions in our lives and sometimes found the visits interesting. After we had lived with friends a few weeks, Daddy would show up and talk to Mother. Then we would all go home again. Daddy might work on one of his inventions for a while and, apparently wouldn't drink. Once, during one of these more harmonious periods, we made exciting plans to go live in the mountains and earn our living prospecting for gold. (Daddy was good at devised grandiose plans to become rich.)

Another disturbing element in our childhood was my maternal grandmother, who divided her time by living with each of her two children. In both families she chose one grandchild upon whom she lavished love and gifts, and regarded the others as enemies. My sister was the recipient of her affection in our family.

Mother would call us together and warn us Gram was coming.

"Try to behave," she would beg us.

My brother and I would regard each other with sudden devotion, forgetting all personal squabbles. We remained united, devising torments for my poor sister, until the day Gram finally returned to my uncle's family. (Our baby sister, nine years younger than I, wasn't yet involved.) Gram's husband, my maternal grandfather, died when I was three, and I never knew him. His children always spoke of him with respect and affection. Housing his family in a covered wagon, he had earned a living as a traveling photographer. When he became older he went off and lived alone in the desert. Considering Gram's sharp, caustic tongue and cantankerous disposition, one might understand his desire to escape. Gram used to intentionally try to embarrass Mother by gleefully smacking her lips over a glass of water, pretending it was gin, whenever the preacher called.

When we were small, we fought and bickered like a bunch of puppies, and Gram scrapped like one of the litter. Daddy, for whom she never had a kind word, usually suffered in silence, but once she must have gone too far, and he told her to leave. She wasn't ready to return to my uncle's house. She put a tent up in the back yard and camped out there until she wore Daddy down with her sarcastic remarks, and he allowed her back into the house.

Today, I can feel compassion for them all, as I try to imagine having to live with my grown children, and sleeping on a cot in the dining room. In her later years, Gram had to work as a practical nurse for what money she had. The day she turned sixty-five, and the State granted her an old-age stipend, she went to bed and stayed there until her death some ten years later.

Mother was a friendly, out going woman, but also tolerant and non-judgmental. Crippled by rheumatoid arthritis since the age of thirty, she was cheerful and affectionate in spite of constant pain. Everyone loved and admired her. She must have had great courage. Anyone believing a mother creates her child's emotional health would have a hard time explaining the difference between my mother and my grandmother.

As teenagers, the highlight of our life was a church summer-camp for which we worked all year to earn the money. One evening at camp, six girls from Ukiah, housed in a cabin, decided to do the most daring, outrageous thing our imaginations could devise. Pulling the blinds and locking the door - we played strip poker! The Methodists running the camp learned of our escapade and announced our disgrace publicly. They stood us up in front of assembly, and everyone prayed we would repent our sins. Such humiliation might have been unbearable if there hadn't been six of us. Together, we just obligingly repented and allowed ourselves to become "saved", creating a wonderful big emotional event for everyone. (Until our poker-playing escapade, everyone at camp had been regarded as already "saved".)

I embraced my salvation enthusiastically, and when I got home, looked around for someone to proselytize. My father had never to my knowledge been to church. At my question of, "Have you considered accepting Christ into your life?", my poor inarticulate father shot me a startled glance and got up and left the house. I was too full of fun to remain preoccupied with religion for long though. (No matter the religion or sect, I never heard of a god known for his sense of humor.) I remember an aunt's evasive answers when I asked why she didn't go to church, but I never had serious doubts about religion until I reached college.

Many people who become skeptical of religious myths and legends turn to materialism and become as zealously evangelical about their newly found "scientific truth" as any religion. They insist the universe is merely the result of accidental processes, without design, plan or purpose—that life consists of nothing but matter and known physical forces, and free will is merely an illusion created by a computer-like mechanism in our head. They argue that if there were any purpose to life, suffering and injustice would not exist. I've always had an instinctive faith that the way the universe is, is the way the universe is supposed to be, and I don't regard injustice and suffering as examples of nature's foul-ups. A perfect society would be incapable of growth, static rather than dynamic. In other words, dead! I suspect Heaven (no suffering) would be too boring for human tolerance, and we would self-destruct. How can I deplore suffering and injustice and still regard them as a normal part of life? So-called logical minds have difficulty with such paradoxes. Agnosticism claims the human mind is incapable of such comprehension, and had served me for many years as a religious label.

The most traumatic event of my childhood happened when I was twenty-two. Some people might be adults at that age, but I was in some ways immature. Mother left my father, again, and came to live with me. She bought a house with the money my brother in the Navy was sending her. When I decided to go to Alaska, I took a bus trip to the town where my father lived to tell him goodbye. We walked out of the busy garage where Daddy worked, and he stood silently, his eyes on the ground, while I explained why I'd come.

"Go away," he said, looking up at me with bitterness. "I'm not interested in where you go. Your mother has been with you for nearly a year, and I haven't heard a word from you."

"I'm sorry, I—"

"Just go away. I don't want to see you again."

He turned and walked away from me. His back and lowered head disappeared into the garage. I stood there a moment, overcome with terrible, confused feelings of anger, shame, guilt and regret. Then I got on the bus and returned to Berkeley. It hadn't occurred to me my father might want to see me after Mother left him. During my college years I'd made trips home several times a year. My father, with problems of his own, never had much to say. Mother was the one who showed affection and expressed interest in our lives.

At the age of twenty-two, I had the rest of my life to sort out my thoughts and feelings, but my last sight of my father was his back disappearing into that garage. Daddy died a few months later and I was left with all the things I might have said to him. Self-centered at that age, I didn't understand much about suffering. So far, my cheerful, optimistic nature had allowed me to sail through life unscathed. As the years passed and I gained understanding, I realized how alone Daddy must have felt. If he hadn't loved us he wouldn't have stayed and tried to earn a living all those years. He never mistreated us; the worst thing he did while drinking was fall down. I remembered incidents that must have been his inhibited way of showing affection.

For instance, my sister once forgot her kitten on a camping trip. Daddy turned the car around and drove fifty miles back into the mountains to search for it. Once, Daddy came home from a fishing trip with a box of interesting pets for us— bats. They escaped and flew all over the house, and it was hours before we got rid of them. None of us, especially Mother, thought they were cute.

I became aware of traits in myself, such as mathematical ability and my nonconformist tendencies, which I felt I'd inherited from my father.

Perhaps seeing his failures helped me to deal with my own nature. Every year that memory of the suffering I inflicted upon my father by my thoughtless concern with my own life has become more painful. How deserted Daddy must have felt. If only I had acquired more wisdom by that age.

I had painful childhood memories all right. I experienced all the violent emotions of childhood: rage, resentment, jealousy and envy, and suffered them consciously, not subconsciously. I suffered shame over my father's drinking. I remembered occasions when I was intentionally dishonest and hurtful, without feeling much guilt. I recalled, after some well-deserved punishment, vivid fantasies of tragically expiring - and then they would all be sorry for the way they had treated me!

On the other hand, I also remembered birthday parties, the circus coming to town, Mother making me a new dress, and hot summer afternoons when we walked two miles for a swim in the river. I remember Daddy coming up with the price of a quart of ice cream on a sweltering summer evening. I can still recall the delicious, cool nights when we all moved our beds into the back yard at the beginning of summer. As a teenager I remember boy friends, picnics, dances, football games and stealing watermelons from farmers' fields. A boxcar load of watermelons was damaged one summer, and we were allowed to steal all we wanted. I have joyful recollections of singing Shine on Harvest Moon or My Gal Sal at the top of our lungs on balmy summer evenings, while chugging down a country lane in a jalopy overflowing with spirited seventeen year olds. I remember laughing until we collapsed at things adults didn't seem to consider funny.

There was the time I sent for travel brochures from magazines in the library. The mailman delivered our mail in a carton for a few weeks. I spent hours of exquisite fantasy in exotic places like Ceylon and Maracaibo and, of course, being rescued from a never-ending series of perils by a stalwart hero on a white horse. (It would be difficult to reach the Seychelles on a horse, and my hero often rode a yacht.) Believing myself to be the only person living a fantasy life, I never admitted to such a pastime. Mother fussed because I put the dustpan in the icebox and the butter in the broom closet. Meanwhile, I floated serenely down the Congo on my yacht. Crocodiles frolicked in the muddy water, and naked pygmies hid behind banana trees along the shore. Tarzan lurked up in the trees, ready to rescue me from perils.

As a child I noticed the lives and families of my friends were not always perfect. Since growing up, I've become aware many of the people I like and respect the most had a more difficult childhood than mine. Although I had never paid much attention to psychology, I had become aware that a number of people claim to have been damaged by a childhood with an alcoholic parent. Nevertheless I was an individual, not a statistic, and I refused to conform to some psychiatric formula. I was determined Dr. Dingle would not talk me into some traumatic childhood I didn't remember experiencing. I continued the dreaded, weekly ordeal of group therapy, but had no intention of discussing my past with a psychologist.

CHAPTER 10

Can the therapist suffer rejection from the patient?

When group therapy ended in the spring, Dr. Dingle announced he was transferring to a hospital in another state and asked us each to his office for a final consultation.

"Tony should continue therapy with Dr. Lavalle," he said, as I warily seated myself across the desk from him, "but you certainly don't need any psychiatric treatment."

What was he up to now?

He gave an unconvincing little laugh, blushed, and looked away from my distrustful scrutiny. Then, fumbling with some papers on his desk, he continued, "In the future, I suggest you come in occasionally with your husband and report Tony's progress to Colonel Mann."

Colonel Mann seemed closer to my own age. I hadn't enjoyed a pink-cheeked young man in his twenties trying to teach me about mother-hood. Maybe I'd get along better with the colonel.

Colonel Mann took a vacation. For a while that summer neither Ike nor I talked to a psychologist, although we continued to take Tony for what they called his play therapy. One day as I waited in the clinic for Tony, Colonel Mann, back from his holiday, came out of his office and spoke to me.

"Tell your husband I'll see him next week at the usual time."

"Do you want me to come too?" The psychologist hesitated as if trying to make up his mind. "Dr. Dingle said—" I began.

"Oh, I suppose you can come along if you want," he finally conceded with exaggerated indifference. Thus, Ike and I began our second year of psychotherapy.

"Tony's prospects are very bright if we all cooperate here," Colonel Mann said at our first meeting. "His future looks bleak if we don't."

I was convinced Tony's future had nothing to do with our psychiatric treatment. Nevertheless, I suppressed my annoyance at the psychologist's authoritative statements. I didn't want him to get angry and say something he couldn't retract, as I suspected Dr. Dingle had. I was still confident I could convince any reasonable person I was a good mother. Perhaps when Colonel Mann realized I was not the type of woman to cause anyone to become abnormal, and certainly not my children, he would then discuss this thing he thought might be wrong with Tony.

"What's wrong with Tony?" I asked Colonel Mann.

"There is nothing physically wrong with him," he answered.

Tony hadn't been given a physical examination. Doctors, I had learned, give many tests to children suspected of mental retardation. Some I'd read of were electroencephalograms, skull X-rays, blood and urine tests and basal metabolism tests. This clinic was part of Letterman Hospital, a large, well equipped, and highly respected facility. Since no one had suggested any such tests, the psychologists must know Tony was not retarded. Doctors appeared to recognize some specific diagnosis, which ruled out retardation.

During the weeks that followed, thinking of something to talk about often became burdensome. Ike and the psychologist sometimes discussed fishing. As the hour drew to a close, we'd wait for the sound of Tony running down the hall from the playroom. Then he'd burst eagerly into the psychologist's office, bright-eyed and grinning with anticipation, looking for his candy.

"The idea is to frustrate Tony-and then reward him," Colonel Mann would explain. The psychologist would put his foot up on the desk so Tony couldn't reach the drawer where candy was kept. Tony did not question the strange ways of psychologists and had single-minded determination about sweets. He cheerfully pushed and pulled on the psychologist, trying to crawl over and under him, until Colonel Mann finally allowed him to get to the candy.

"See, I'm making myself important to Tony by giving him candy. Now Mommy must think of ways to make herself important," the psychologist would say. "Then Tony will stop rejecting Mommy."

"Tony doesn't reject me."

"We're going to teach Mommy to understand Tony," he promised, ignoring my protest.

"I understand Tony pretty well," I said.

"He wouldn't act as he does if you understood him! When Mommy learns to understand Tony, he'll act like other children. Sometimes I wonder if Mommy comprehends how different Tony is. Why, he doesn't even compare favorably with most two year olds."

I was painfully aware. Tony was still in diapers. Shortly before his fifth birthday, we had persuaded him to urinate in the toilet by feeding him full of watermelon. Then the whole family cooperated to entertain him, as we stood him in the bathroom without trousers. When he finally urinated into the toilet, we cheered. Tony laughed. After that urinating into things became a game to him. We had no success with bowel movements.

"Perhaps Tony doesn't think highly enough of himself to want to give away part of his body," suggested Colonel Mann.

I had recently read a psychiatric theory claiming man's first love, even before love of mother, was love of his own excrement. I suspected some people might consider such a theory an obscenity if anyone but a psychiatrist uttered it. Nevertheless, I resolved not to argue. I tried to sit quietly each week and endure Colonel Mann's psychology.

As Tony's fifth birthday neared, I realized he would not be mature enough to attend kindergarten and I looked for a nursery school. One turned out to be a ballet class for four year olds. Tony would have considered ballet a preposterous activity, and we laughed at the thought of independent, super-masculine Tony in a ballet class. However, no nursery school would accept a child with a problem. They were especially suspicious when I said Tony wasn't retarded, but I didn't know what was wrong with him. At a public-school, county-run nursery school for retarded children, I tried to describe Tony to the teacher. She suggested he sounded antisocial. She pointed to a good-looking little boy who sat laughing to himself. He was a bundle of constant motion, playing with blocks with one hand and furiously twirling something with the other.

"That little boy lives in a world of his own," she said. "He's schizo-phrenic."

We asked Dr. Lavalle to mail a report about Tony to Marin County schools. Then Ike and I went to discuss the possibility of Tony attending the class. Dr. Lavalle's report lay on the desk before the school psychologist. I looked longingly at the folder. I wished we—Tony's parents, were permitted to read what doctors and psychologists wrote about our child.

"Tony doesn't qualify for this program," explained the school psychologist. "He's not mentally retarded. Children like your son are smart enough; they are emotionally immature."

The class for retarded children would have been good for Tony. Life would have been easier for all of us during the next four years if he could have attended school. We should have fought for his acceptance.

Maybe, like many people, we harbored a suspicion retardation might be contagious. Indeed, it was commonly believed IQ scores were culturally induced. We were probably relieved not to expose Tony to the harmful influence of a class of subnormal children. I did feel a secret triumph at having Tony's lack of retardation stated so officially, confirming my belief that doctors recognized some specific diagnosis. Finally, I found a nursery school. The teacher was a compassionate woman, and my ardent gratitude seemed to compensate her for any extra trouble Tony caused. I promised to stay by the telephone, ready to come for him if he ever became a problem.

While passing out cupcakes for PTA at Guy's and Sherry's school one afternoon I heard of another unusual child. I got the mother's name and phoned her. We talked a long time and discovered our children had similarities. Both were slow to talk, toilet train and learn the things children accomplish before school age. Both liked to play by themselves. Her experience became painful when her pediatrician suggested she and her husband weren't really happy. After listening to her doctor repeat that suggestion for several months, she and her husband weren't very happy. In fact, they were constantly at each other's throats over what to do with the child. They finally took him to a March-of-Dimes, birth-defects clinic, which diagnosed him as suffering from minimal brain damage, or neurological dysfunction. The parents were told their child had an excellent chance of living a normal life. There was no medical treatment for the condition.

"Obtaining a positive diagnosis was a relief," the mother said. I was aware of the agony of living with an unknown. "They said Eric is artistic," she added.

"So is Tony," I said. "I never heard of anyone calling that an abnormality, though."

I envied Eric's mother her peace of mind. Nevertheless, I couldn't imagine Tony's diagnosis being neurological damage. He had a hypersensitive nervous system, and his reactions were faster than those of normal people. His coordination was exceptional. He could turn his tricycle upside down and balance himself on the pedals while trying to rotate them.

           *   *   *

Ike's and my weekly talks with Colonel Mann dragged on. I hated the uncomfortable silences that sometimes developed. I struggled against an urge to blurt out something—anything—to fill them. I suspected psychologists might use silence as a tool to induce patients to blurt out confession of some neurosis, but Ike was usually able to think of some comment to save me from such a fate. One day no one could think of anything to say. Finally, Colonel Mann said to me, "I don't know what your differences with Dr. Dingle were. Maybe they were just philosophical."

I felt I'd avoided philosophical discussions. It sounded like a glib dismissal of that entire, awful year of group therapy.

"This has been hard on my wife," Ike said. "I've tried to explain it was a probing to find out if there *could* be a problem in our family."

I remained silent. Ike was an admirer of my emotional stability, and felt it must be obvious to the psychologist. He didn't fully understand how offended I felt by all this probing. I wondered if he'd feel such tolerant understanding if the probing had been directed at him.

"And of course you take an especially close look at the mother when you suspect emotional problems," Ike continued, always able to understand someone else's point of view.

I didn't expect an apology. However, I felt that, at the very least, I deserved an acknowledgment that no one had unearthed any sinister flaw in my character. The psychologist was staring glumly out the window. The silence dragged on.

The psychologist wasn't agreeing with Ike, I realized. He still believed my emotional maltreatment had made Tony abnormal! Sitting through these two awful years of psychology had accomplished nothing.

Something in me snapped. Or maybe it wasn't a sudden change; perhaps I'd been gradually losing my fear of psychologists. In any case, I was startled to suddenly hear myself boldly challenge Colonel Mann,

"You used the term mentally retarded last week. If you suspect retardation, why hasn't Tony been given tests?"

"The term mentally retarded doesn't necessarily mean mentally defective," the psychologist explained, ignoring the hostility in my voice. "Tony's development is retarded, but we can tell by looking he's not mentally defective. The hands and feet of defective children sometimes develop differently, for instance." I wondered why doctors bothered with tests if psychologists could determine retardation by looking? "Besides," the psychologist added, "we'll soon be able to give Tony an intelligence test."

"Intelligence test," I repeated scornfully.

The psychologist looked annoyed. I had no particular criticism of IQ tests. Frustrated by months of trying to make conversation, I was exploding. In fact, it was a turning point in my life, a dramatic change in my reaction to people. From that day I began to shed the overpowering feeling of intimidation I felt in the presence of doctors—or anyone else for that matter.

"For over a year I've listened to you psychologists accuse me of horrible things. Now I want to know about those other children like Tony. What happened when they grew up?" I demanded.

"You are right," the psychologist agreed, ignoring my question. "We've said harsh things to you. It was necessary. We had to make Mommy do something about Tony."

What gave him such a right? I was also fed up with listening to the psychologist call me "Mommy".

"It's important to remember we are all trying to help Tony," Ike cautioned, startled by such an aggressive manner from his usually diffident wife.

I glared at him.

"I don't know how to talk to psychologists," I said. "Other people just say what they mean."

"Don't you think I mean what I say?" the psychologist asked.

"I never know what you are up to. Most of the time you seem to be trying to maneuver me, hoping your psychology will have some effect upon me."

"Well, now—" Ike said.

"Oh, we've given up hope of having any effect upon you," Colonel Mann said. "In fact, it's a damned shame how much time and money we've wasted on you without accomplishing anything, isn't it?"

I scowled at him and continued,

"No one will answer my question about what might happen to Tony. I'll bet the truth is all those withdrawn children, or whatever they are called, grew up all right."

The psychologist shrugged.

"Dr. Dingle was willing to use anything short of a rubber hose to make me admit I wasn't emotionally involved with my children," I said. "If something terrible happens to children like Tony, he'd have been delighted to tell me."

"Maybe they grew up all right, but maybe they didn't grow up to be desirable people."

"I'm not asking what you think might have happened to them. I'm asking what did happen to them—if you even know."

"Yes" Ike agreed, "what did—"

"Besides," I continued, "I've decided what you consider desirable, and what I consider desirable, might be two different things. Who do you psychologists think you are, anyway, to decide what people should and shouldn't be?"

"Would you consider it desirable if Tony grew up to steal cars?"

"I'll buy him a c—" Ike tried to offer.

"I don't for one moment think he will steal cars," I said. "Maybe he is just going to grow up to be like me. You might not approve, but it's none of your damned business."

"Yes! Except you talk!"

Then he added under his breath, "unfortunately."

"I have an appointment," Ike muttered, glancing toward the door.

"Is Tony psychotic?" I demanded.

"That word is difficult to define."

"Do you consider him schizophrenic?"

"We considered it!"

"And what conclusion did you come to?"

"Well, we don't like to use labels."

"Does or doesn't the term childhood schizophrenia apply to Tony?" I persisted.

"Yes!" the psychologist shouted.

There was a moment of stunned silence.

"We have to leave," Ike said. "I'm late for an appointment."

Ike never spoke impolitely to anyone, and he'd never heard me attack anyone so belligerently. He obviously wanted to escape from this embarrassing melee. The psychologist had been about to continue angrily, but stopped and looked at Ike.

"We have accomplished one thing for you in therapy," he said. "We've pointed out a difference of opinion seems to exist between you and your wife."

"My husband and I are capable of living with differences of opinion," I snapped. "We don't try to stuff our beliefs down each other's throats."

Ike and I got Tony from the playroom and left. In the waiting room I noticed people eye us with curiosity. At times our therapy had probably become so loud everyone heard.

In the car I accused Ike,

"I suppose you agree I need a psychologist to tell me how to treat the children?"

"I didn't say that."

"You said—"

"Don't start telling me what I said. I didn't even get in a word."

"That damned psychologist said Tony hasn't grown up because of me, and you didn't disagree."

"I didn't hear him say that!"

"It's what he really meant!"

"How the hell do you know what he really meant?"

"The Goddamn psy—"

Tony, frightened, reached over from the back seat and tried to hold his hand over my mouth. Ike and I stopped shouting and drove home in smoldering silence. During the next week Ike and I erupted into argument whenever we tried to discuss Tony. I had come across the term childhood schizophrenia and had read that it was unrelated to adult schizophrenia. I'd read some children outgrow childhood schizophrenia, but had been unable to find out what happened to those who didn't.

When we returned to the clinic the following week, Colonel Mann apologized.

"I'm afraid I said things I didn't mean last week."

"And I'm sorry I became so angry," I said. "I know your intentions were good, but I have loathed every minute of this therapy."

Ike asked again if the term childhood schizophrenia applied to Tony.

"Yes. But remember, there are different degrees of it," Colonel Mann cautioned.

I felt a pang of fear. I wished calling Tony schizophrenic were one of the things the psychologist hadn't meant to say. Even a mild case of schizophrenia sounded terrifying to me.

Then Colonel Mann turned to me.

"I've stated that if Mommy wants to know the cause of Tony's illness, she must look to herself. However, I want to emphasize again I do not blame Mommy for what has happened to her child."

Now that's big of you, I was tempted to retort. I knew psychologists felt smug about not blaming mothers who don't love their children. Dr. Dingle sat unperturbed while some of the women in the group expressed resentment and hostility toward their families. The only thing that really angered him was my insistence that I didn't have any such feelings.

"You are entitled to your opinion. But as Tony's mother, I know he isn't suffering from emotional problems," I argued.

"Tony certainly does have emotional problems," protested the psychologist. "We wouldn't treat him here at the clinic if he didn't."

"Tony is obviously a happy child," Ike pointed out.

"Don't let that happy smile on his face fool you," the psychologist said. "There is absolutely no doubt Tony either is, or has been, extremely unhappy."

"There are doctors who disagree with you," I objected.

"I never heard of any. That civilian psychiatrist you went to last year sure got Tony's number fast. He phoned and asked about this autistic child we were treating."

The psychologist was still talking, but I wasn't listening.

Autistic! I'll bet that's what the mother I spoke to on the phone said. Her little boy, Eric, was autistic—not artistic. Maybe Tony had more in common with her child than I'd thought.

It was nearly two years since I'd first taken Tony to a doctor, and this was the first time I became aware of the term "autistic". Psychologists had reason for reluctance to use it to parents. With the phrase "not emotionally involved", they were trying to state everything euphemistically, while psychiatric journals stated bluntly autism was caused by maternal rejection. When psychologists did begin using the term, parents of autistic children, some of whom were themselves doctors, read psychiatric journals and they vigorously protested such psychiatric theories.

CHAPTER 11

Do doctors close ranks when challenged?

That evening I begged Ike to quit the psychologists. I wanted to take Tony to the Birth-defects Clinic, where that mother on the phone told me her little boy, Eric, was diagnosed autistic and minimal brain damaged.

"Remember," Ike cautioned, "that clinic offered no treatment."

"You've seen a sample of psychotherapy. Surely you don't believe it's going to cure Tony of anything. Think what a relief it would be to find someone who would discuss his diagnosis." Ike agreed.

"Why do you want to take Tony there?" the psychologist objected when we told him. "We've already told you there is nothing physically wrong with him."

"But you've never given him a physical examination," I said.

He frowned, but otherwise ignored the point. "They might not be willing to see Tony when they learn we've been treating you for nearly two years," he said.

What a silly notion! Did he think the psychiatric clinic owned us? In any case, we could try. Finally, seemingly resigned that he couldn't dissuade us, the psychologist said,

"Children like your son get upset if their routine is disturbed. It would be unwise to interrupt his play therapy. We hope you'll continue bringing Tony to the clinic, although you should probably stop therapy while seeing another doctor."

We thanked him. Maybe we were naive not to realize we should break all ties with the Child Guidance Clinic before consulting another doctor. Nevertheless, in this case it probably would not have mattered. Unbeknownst to us, autism was the subject of widespread research. Many doctors considered scientific research more important than patients and cooperated with each other. In fact, in those days the medical profession felt justified in conducting research on patients without their knowledge or consent.

Colonel Mann claimed he was unable to refer Tony to the Birth-Defects Clinic himself, but told us the name of the woman in charge, a well-known pediatrician who also had a private practice. He suggested we make appointment with her to get Tony an evaluation at that clinic.

When we met the new doctor at her office, her common-sense manner invited confidence. She was older than I. At the time she became a doctor, there were no affirmative action programs, and I knew she must have been an exceptional woman to finish medical school. I felt her outstanding reputation must surely be justified.

"It's not that I don't believe in emotional problems," I told her. "I don't believe emotional problems are causing Tony's slow development."

"The trouble with psychiatry is they have misinterpreted Freud," she said.

"Yes," I agreed, inclined to agree with anyone who suggested psychiatry might have misinterpreted something.

She examined Tony briefly and then commented, "Tony may not be an Einstein, but I see no reason why he can't be educated to lead a happy, useful life. Before doing anything else, however, let's evaluate your son at the Birth-Defects Clinic and determine how much he is perceiving." She gave us an appointment.

The Birth-Defects Clinic apparently had some test to determine how much children perceived. If perceiving meant noticing things, I suspected Tony did more of it than most people, but this was the first doctor to suggest Tony wasn't extremely bright. If he was retarded, surely it was time someone told us! Loss of faith in recognized authority is a frightening experience. Most people, reluctant to endure such insecurity, stubbornly resist liberation. I had managed to live without an officially recognized religion, but was clinging to my faith in scientific medicine. This pediatrician seemed straightforward and unimpressed with psychotherapy as a treatment for illness. I desperately wanted to trust a doctor and was prepared to believe whatever she said.

The pediatrician had suggested doctors and psychologists were misinterpreting Freud. (I suppose declaring him to be just plain wrong would have been unthinkable in those days.) I had tried again to read Freud but found little in his obscure, wordy formulas that felt relevant to me. Freud insisted the most likely cause of neuroses was an infant witnessing the human sex act. He once had a patient, Princess Marie Bonaparte, so emotionally messed up he was convinced she must have seen someone copulate when she was an infant.

"Impossible," she assured him. "My mother died soon after my birth, and I was raised by my father and grandmother. No sex took place on our estate."

Freud continued to insist only witnessing the human sex act could cause such monumental neurosis, and she investigated the circumstances of her infancy. When she interrogated one of her father's former grooms, he confessed to an affair with her wet nurse before Marie was a year old. Freud felt satisfied that her injured psyche was thus explained.

I thought of my son Guy's attitude toward sex. When about six, after watching the squirrels in the yard, he asked,

"How do you tell a mommy squirrel from a daddy squirrel?"

"Personally, I can't," I answered, not eager to get into such a discussion with a six-year-old.

"I guess squirrels must be able to tell the difference, even if people can't," he mused. "Otherwise you'd have two daddy squirrels sitting around in the same tree, each waiting for the other one to have a baby squirrel."

I didn't correct him. Our family had all the inhibitions of our time. Unbelievable in today's society, we didn't even use the word penis. We called it a whot-tossie. I was relieved this new pediatrician didn't seem inclined to go into such matters

(Today everyone watches sex simulated on television, and the only effect it seems to have, on adults or infants, is slight boredom. Present-day sufferers of what Freud called hysteria usually feel compelled, with the help of therapists, to develop multiple personalities and "remember" something more lurid, such as incest or Satanic ritual abuse.)

While awaiting our appointment at the Birth-Defects Clinic, I tried to learn the meanings of the terms, *autism* and *childhood schizophrenia*. I found psychiatric journals at the University of California library. In 1943, Leo Kanner, a psychiatrist at Johns Hopkins Hospital in Baltimore, described a few young children with startling and unique characteristics. He called the condition *early infantile autism*. Although retarded in their mental development, the children appeared bright and alert. Their coordination was good, and sometimes superior. From infancy they showed aversion to being held or cuddled; they were not responsive to people and did not form emotional attachments to anyone. They displayed an obsessive desire for their environment to remain the same. Such children became upset, for instance, if the furniture was rearranged. Many had unusual musical talent and prodigious memories for such things as numbers. One child could quickly memorize entire scores of operas. They had little ability for abstract thinking. Some did not talk, and those who spoke were often echolaic, parroting back whatever was said to them. Their parents were highly educated, and reported by psychiatrists to be "cold".

Some of this described Tony; some did not. But as I read psychiatric journals, I found many children called autistic whom the description did not seem to fit. There were volumes of discussions about such children's defective psyches, and the defective psyches of their parents. Like me, most mothers of autistic children were reported to resist psychiatric treatment, an attitude psychiatrists viewed with greaat suspicion. I couldn't find a definition of *childhood schizophrenia*. A group of children with widely varying characteristics might be called *autistic*, and as far as I could determine, did not differ from other groups who were called *schizophrenic* or *disturbed*. At a large, busy, technical-book store in San Francisco, I stood and searched through the newest medical tomes on the shelves, but was unable to find definitions.

My medical literature search was interrupted by the unexpected arrival of Ike's overseas orders. We had forgotten that Ike, still a few years before retirement, could be transferred. New assignments had once seemed exciting. Now, such an undertaking loomed as an overwhelming complication. Ike wrote the Department of the Army, requesting a delay, and asked Colonel Mann to write a letter of endorsement. Colonel Mann agreed to write the letter but didn't show it to Ike, sending it directly to the Personnel Department. We wondered if Colonel Mann had stated Tony's diagnosis. Knowing a sergeant in the Personnel Department, Ike managed to obtain a copy. There was an uncertain look on his face as he gave it to me. As I read it, I understood, for I found the language offensive. Colonel Mann's letter read:

1. Anthony Vandegrift, five-year-old dependent son of Sgt. and Mrs. Vandegrift, has been under treatment at this child guidance clinic since May 1961. Presenting symptoms were those of an autistic child in that Anthony was socially withdrawn, fearful of people, essentially nonverbal, behaviorally inappropriate and indifferent to efforts at socialization. Difficulties were made apparent to the mother who nevertheless attempted to deny the severity of the boy's problem, which began at the age of three, during the father's assignment to Greenland for 13 months.

2. Treatment was initiated with the mother and son with only limited effect until the father's return 15 months ago. Since his return to the family, and with the aid of parental counseling in the Child Guidance clinic, there has been a slow but steady improvement in Anthony's adjustment, most apparent in increased verbalization, response to parental requests, and security in new situations. Anthony's change from indifference to interest in the world and people has been in large measure due to the presence of the father, who more than the mother has understood his son's problems and special needs.

3. Sgt. Vandegrift is now subject to overseas assignment to Germany where suitable educational and treatment facilities for emotionally disturbed children, like his son, are not available. Should the father go overseas alone, however, his son would be left without a principal source of security, understanding and model for learning in the family.

I never dreamed the medical profession indulged in such petty dishonesty. Much of the misrepresentation might be blamed on lack of objectivity. Psychologists see what they want to see. However, it was blatantly untrue that I had started treatment "with limited effect" before Ike's return from Greenland. Perhaps Colonel Mann described me as unfit to be left alone with Tony only to help delay Ike's overseas orders. Even so, I found it difficult to feel grateful. Several years later I managed to get my hands on Tony's medical records. They were sealed, but I carefully pried out the staples and covertly read another report from the Child Guidance Clinic. That report was signed by some doctor I'd never met. That doctor claimed Tony had been very ill when he first came to the clinic. He wrote that psychotherapy had helped him improve, but each time Tony returned to the family situation, he regressed. The doctor stated that as soon as this became apparent to the mother, she suddenly withdrew the child from treatment. *(How on earth did he define the word suddenly?)*

I had no idea why this unknown doctor should say something so far from the truth. It sounded almost vindictive. The report said they had diagnosed Tony as autistic but later changed their diagnosis to child-hood schizophrenia. (Without ever informing us?) In the years after we quit the Child Guidance Clinic, we were never able to free ourselves from these psychiatric reports. Every time we consulted a new doctor, or tried to enroll Tony in a school, reports were required from everyone who had ever treated him. It was frustrating to know such defamatory distortions followed us. We couldn't refute them without admitting we had read them. Parents were never permitted to read what doctors and psychologists wrote about them or their children.

I've found Army medicine to be comparable to civilian practice. The people we dealt with were not bad psychologists. They were well-inten-tioned men zealously promoting bad theories. Other parents of autistic children were receiving similar treatment in civilian psychiatric clinics during that period. I know of several who managed to get a glimpse of their children's psychiatric reports. They were equally shocked at how psychologists can malign parents with little regard for facts. Psychologists have no means of judging if parents reject their children. They can't even distinguish a healthy psyche from a damaged one. Therapists might be inclined to regard anyone who disliked therapy as "cold."

Because of Colonel Mann's letter, the Army canceled Ike's overseas orders. For that, we were relieved. We continued taking Tony to Dr. Lavalle. The next week as Tony and I were leaving the clinic after his play therapy, I looked up and saw Colonel Mann come out of his office. He started across the waiting room toward me, a huge smile on his face, suggesting a friendliness I viewed with suspicion. I realized I should be grateful to him for writing the letter, but how could I pretend gratitude toward a man who had described me as such a terrible mother?

Oh, let Ike thank him, I decided. Grabbing Tony by the hand, I turned and hurried out of the clinic, leaving the psychologist standing in the middle of the waiting room.

We took Tony for his evaluation at the March-of-Dimes clinic. Specialists observed Tony, and a psychiatric social worker questioned Ike and me. Although she and I were to meet a few years later under ominous circumstances, at that time the social worker seemed like a nice lady. Ike and I, desperate to trust someone, answered all her questions. After the examination the pediatrician in charge of the clinic told us many tests and many trips to the clinic might be necessary to diagnose Tony. She asked us to sign a release, allowing her to send for Tony's records from the Child Guidance Clinic.

The pediatrician had expressed skepticism about psychiatry, claiming Freud had been misinterpreted. Surely she had enough common sense not to be influenced by whatever the psychologists said about us. We signed the release.

The following week, before we'd taken Tony for any further tests, the pediatrician in charge of the clinic phoned and asked us to return to her private office where we'd first met her. She was nervously looking through Tony's records when we arrived.

"The government is doing more every day for the retarded," she declared. "In a few years, we'll have some kind of guardianship for these children. The way things are now, the children grow up and commit some crime for which they aren't really responsible. Then the state demands they be sent to the gas chamber. It's a ridiculous system."

What was she implying? Death in the gas chamber was a shocking possibility for any doctor to mention to the parents of a five-year-old child. This pediatrician was a well-known doctor, and obviously a kind, intelligent, compassionate woman. Such a remark seemed out of character. *Did she, for some reason feel obligated to try to frighten us?*

"Is Tony mentally retarded?" I asked, trying to recover from the shock of her statement…

"What does that term mean?" the doctor countered. "Recently I spoke before a group of parents. Most of them thought mental retardation meant mongolism. Oh, your child is not mentally defective. We can tell that by looking."

During our first visit she had felt unable to determine retardation by looking. She'd planned to give Tony tests. What had happened? She had seemed so reasonable and candid before. *Could her change of attitude be caused by whatever the Child Guidance Clinic had written?*

"I guess you don't know Tony's diagnosis," I said, struggling with a wrenching feeling of disappointment.

"No. He could be emotionally disturbed," she said. "I strongly urge you to continue psychiatric treatment." During our first visit, she hadn't believed emotional problems could cause retarded development. Then, as she watched me fighting back tears, her grim expression seemed to melt a little, and she added sympathetically,

"It could be in his genes—or his brain. We know so little about the human brain."

"What about childhood schizophrenia?" I asked.

"Who knows why some people break down under conditions others survive?" She turned impatiently to Ike. "You've been through the war, Sergeant. You must realize we don't know."

"Is Tony schizophrenic?" I asked again.

The pediatrician hesitated. Again I caught a look of sympathy in her face. "Pseudo schizophrenia, I call it," she finally said apologetically.

"That term autism—"

"Oh that doesn't mean anything," the doctor said hastily. "Just that some children relate to people differently."

"Is Tony brain damaged?" I asked. This same pediatrician had told that mother on the phone her little boy was minimal brain damaged and autistic.

"If you ask a neurologist, he'll say these children are all brain damaged. If you ask a psychiatrist, he'll say they are emotionally disturbed."

Then she muttered, almost to herself, "Late developers, that's what I call them."

I sat, numbed, and held Tony on my lap. The doctor talked some more to Ike, but I sank into a state of dazed defeat. Colonel Mann had suggested other doctors might refuse to see Tony when they found out the Child Guidance Clinic had treated us for two years. I had considered his suggestion ridiculous, but apparently he was right. The pediatrician was acting as though the psychologists did exert some mysterious ownership over us. For some reason, she was refusing to complete Tony's evaluation at the Birth-Defects Clinic.

The next day when I took Tony for his play therapy, I was still suffering a bleak, heavy feeling of despair. We seemed so helpless against a united, all- powerful medical profession. It had been a couple of months since I ran off and left Colonel Mann standing in the middle of the waiting room. He hadn't tried to speak to me again. Since then we nodded warily to each other when we happened to meet around the clinic. On this day however, as I was getting Tony, I glanced up and saw Colonel Mann again come out of his office. He started toward me with that big smile plastered all over his face.

Why was he coming at me on this dreadful day? The pediatrician hadn't wasted time, had she! She must have immediately phoned and assured the psychologist she was sending us back with a stern warning to continue psychiatric treatment.

In frozen panic I stared at the psychologist as he strode toward me. I had summoned the courage to stand up to him on that one occasion,. but I was still inclined to avoid confrontations when possible. Before Colonel Mann reached my side of the waiting room, I managed to recover from my paralysis. I snatched Tony by the hand and yanked him out the door with me, making another escape.

Colonel Mann didn't try to catch me again. He phoned Ike's office and asked him to come to the clinic. Dr. Lavalle was in the office with Colonel Mann. They made it clear that they had no intention of continuing to see

Tony every week unless they also had an opportunity to "help" his mother. As Dr. Dingle had done the year before, Colonel Mann was transferring to a hospital in another state. Ike mentioned I sometimes complained that Dr. Lavalle, the only psychologist who spent time with Tony, had never spoken to us. Ike suggested I might be willing to talk to him.

Colonel Mann had seemed upset at the meeting, Ike reported. Slamming his hat on his head, he had stalked out of the clinic. Then he had returned in confusion to replace his white coat with his uniform jacket

"We do seem to have an even more disastrous effect upon psychologists than they have on us," I commented dejectedly to Ike. So far both psychologists who tried to give me therapy had fled the state. Tony's psychologist had always seemed pleasant, and I was still naively confident I could convince psychologist I didn't need any psychiatric treatment. I agreed to talk to Dr. Lavalle.

CHAPTER 12

A mommy doll, a daddy doll and a baseball bat

Tony had his sixth birthday. Summer passed, and Colonel Mann had transferred away from the clinic before arrangements were made for us to again begin weekly talks, this time with Dr. Lavalle, Tony's psychologist.

"I believe...Tony is of at least...average intelligence," he said at our first meeting, beginning our third year of therapy. He spoke slowly and deliberately, weighing each word and continuing to convey the impression of reticence we'd felt for the past two years. "And I feel certain within a couple of years..." He seemed to be searching for words.

"That Tony will catch up with children his age?" I finished impatiently for him.

Dr. Lavalle nodded thoughtfully.

"I disagree with your theory that Tony's slow development is caused by something in his environment," I said apologetically. Feeling no dislike toward this psychologist, maybe I could establish some kind of honest relationship with him.

"You don't know what my opinions are," he corrected me.

If he was going to keep his opinions secret how could we have honest discussion? Wary of more confrontations however, I remained silent.

Tony's play therapy had been cut short earlier that day when Dr. Lavalle phoned Ike to come for him. The psychologist reported Tony had refused— for the past few weeks—to go into the playroom. He preferred to play out in the busy waiting room.

"I can't keep up with him out there," the psychologist said. "He's all over the place and into everything. Today I put my foot down."

"It's hard to keep up with Tony," I agreed. For some time I'd wanted to discuss Tony's teeth with a doctor, and explained I feared he had cavities in his baby teeth.

"You might ask a dentist about it," the psychologist said. "Today I told Tony he could go into the playroom, stay out in the hall, or even go outside if he wanted. But I can't explore his emotions in the waiting room among all those people."

Explore Tony's emotions! They'd always called whatever Tony did at the clinic play therapy.

"One has to be firm with Tony," I said. "I try not to give him orders I can't enforce. About Tony's teeth though, I don't think a dentist could get his hand in Tony's mouth."

"He'd never get it back out with all five fingers attached," Ike added.

"I don't know. You might mention the problem to a dentist," the psychologist said. "Today I explained to Tony exactly what I expect of him. I believe he desperately needs this direction in his life."

"Reasoning isn't effective with Tony yet," Ike said. "You have our permission to paddle him, if you think that might help."

"I'm concerned about Tony's teeth," I continued, "because he sometimes screams for no apparent reason. Sometimes he knocks his head against a wall. His screams might be in anger or frustration, but Tony would be unable to tell us if he were in pain."

"It would probably be a good idea to get his teeth fixed," the psychologist agreed. "I don't disapprove of spanking. I even spank my own children. But Tony is old enough to reason with. Today I explained to him, reasonably and simply, how he must behave if he wants to continue coming to the clinic. He craves this structure in his life."

If play therapy was beginning to bore Tony, I doubted the psychologist would get him into the playroom by reasoning. Tony knew his own mind, and I'd never been able to talk him into anything. The medical profession seemed uninterested in any of our real problems, and I gave up trying to discuss Tony's teeth.

The next week when I brought Tony to the clinic, I waited to see whether he would go into the playroom, or if the psychologist would send him home again. Tony had a contented little smile on his face, for he now felt at home around the clinic. He took the psychologist's hand and walked down the hall with him. Tony looked boyish and adorable, his tattered sweater hanging from his shoulders. When they reached the playroom door, Tony stopped. The psychologist bent over and spoke to him. Tony laughed and stamped his little foot rebelliously. He turned and ran back up the hall, watching over his shoulder to see if Dr. Lavalle followed.

"Unless you go into the playroom like a good boy, you'll have to go home," the psychologist warned, following Tony back to the waiting room.

Tony gave a squeal of laughter and darted behind the reception counter. He stood peeking impishly out at the psychologist with a crooked little grin on his face. His eyes sparkled mischievously, and he obviously hoped the psychologist would chase him .Dr. Lavalle sent him home. Tony was still smiling enigmatically as we left, causing me to wonder about his "craving for structure".

That afternoon Ike and I went for our appointment with Dr. Lavalle.

"I was startled last week to hear you speak of trying to explore Tony's emotions," I said. "I can't believe he talks enough to discuss anything that complicated."

"Tony has definite emotions," Dr. Lavalle insisted. He hesitated, and then continued cautiously, "Tony has strong feelings…about both of you. One day I gave him a mama doll and a daddy doll…"

I had read enough psychology books to know a common method of diagnosing a child's hostility toward his parents was to hand him a mama doll, a daddy doll and a baseball bat.

"Tony threw the dolls on the floor…" the psychologist continued.

I tried to conceal my horror.

Then he took a baseball bat…"

His pause hung heavy in the silence.

Get on with it! What did Tony do?

"…then…Tony beat on a chair with the baseball bat," Dr. Lavalle finished in a hushed tone.

I fell back in my chair with relief, and let out the breath I'd been holding. The hostile children I'd read about beat on the dolls. I knew Tony's only interest in dolls would be trying to take them apart. He would enjoy whacking anything with a baseball bat. Tony was remarkably unsusceptible to suggestion, and even urging him to beat on the dolls would probably not have been effective.

"Tony doesn't feel any suppressed hostility toward us," I assured Dr. Lavalle. "He's like a happy little two year old. All two year olds love their parents."

"Maybe you don't allow him to express his feelings openly," the psychologist said.

"If only Tony would start using the toilet," Ike said. "Those diapers bother me more than anything." Ike appeared unconcerned Tony might have some secret desire to hit him over the head with a baseball bat.

"Our television broke last week," I said. "I didn't have the nerve to tell the repairman I'd caught Tony peeing into the back of it."

"And he did it while Dr. Kildare was on," Ike joked. "I wonder if that has any sinister significance?"

The psychologist frowned, apparently failing to find humor in Ike's comment. "It might indicate some of Tony's feelings toward doctors," he said stiffly.

"Tony didn't mean anything by it," I tried to assure him. "He pees into everything these days if I don't watch him. He's always trying to extinguish the pilot light on the furnace."

The psychologist looked unconvinced. He was obviously still a little hurt about Tony's hostile feelings. Ike and I went home laughing about it. Our sense of humor was wearing thin however. Before the evening was over we had another argument about psychiatry. Dr. Lavalle had tried to convince us we weren't strict enough with Tony. The next week he tried to convince us we were too strict. Besides, Tony wasn't even getting his play therapy; the psychologist sent him home each week for not cooperating. Under such circumstances I saw no reason for Ike and me to continue those tedious sessions at the clinic. Ike agreed.

The next week I took Tony to the clinic to give him one more chance. Secretly, I hoped he'd be as uncooperative as the week before. I watched as Dr. Lavalle told Tony "firmly and reasonably" he must go into the playroom. I concealed my satisfaction at Tony's attempts to tease the psychologist. I felt light headed with relief when Dr. Lavalle told Tony he must go home. I thanked the psychologist for being Tony's friend for the past two years. "We aren't coming to the clinic any more," I told him.

A look of alarm flickered across the psychologist's face. Then he conceded, "This treatment is voluntary."

"Yes," I agreed uneasily.

Taking Tony's hand, I turned to go. *Would they actually allow us to leave?* Fearful someone might call me back, I found myself walking faster, pulling Tony down the hall at a run. People in the waiting room stared as we rushed across the room and out the door of the clinic. With pounding heart, I shoved Tony into the car and sped out of the parking lot. I didn't slow down until I noticed a police car. I could imagine the suspicion with which a patrolman might regard me, if as an excuse for speeding, I claimed I was making an escape from a psychiatric clinic.

Thus we "suddenly" quit the psychologists. When we first went to the clinic, therapy wasn't yet such a pervasive part of our culture as it is today, and Ike and I were ignorant about it's nature and purpose. I'd since decided many of the formulas of psychology sounded silly and simplistic. Nevertheless, child psychiatry was an esteemed branch of the medical profession, and Ike had trouble believing doctors could be so wrong. I wanted to do everything possible to help Tony, and that included everything Ike thought might help. Those were the reasons we endured the ordeal for over two years.

I realize some unhappy people find therapy helpful. (I'm still not sure why a degree in psychology should enable someone to determine proper thinking.) For us, however, leaving the psychologists felt as though we had been suffering from a toothache, and weren't aware of how much it hurt until the pain ceased. In spite of our continued fear over Tony's future, I felt ten pounds lighter and ten years younger. Ike had some leave coming. In celebration, we took the children camping in Mexico. Feeling capable of anything now the psychologists were out of my life, I quit smoking.

CHAPTER 13

Can resentment feel like mental illness?

In spite of his increasing differences from other children, I was never able to snuff out a secret belief that Tony might grow up to be normal. Doctors consistently declared him to be extremely bright. He didn't look or act retarded; he was always busy trying to satisfy his monumental curiosity; and it was hard to think of a child as delightfully independent as Tony growing up to be helpless. Had I fully accepted Tony's retardation, I would have grieved. Then the whole family would have recovered and gone on with our lives, doing our best for Tony and for the rest of the family. Most people managed to accept the blows fate dealt them— a disability or death of a loved one. However, each time Tony was denied a service or admission to a school, the feeling of being personally mistreated by some doctor or psychologist plunged me into a malignant pit of anger and resentment. I could understand how patients who are persuaded by therapists to "remember" an unhappy childhood might well find the pain so destructive they feel mentally ill.

I must not take doctors personally, I told myself, as I struggeled against the way anger and resentment made me feel. Forty years experience had taught me people didn't usually take some mysterious, instant dislike to me. Doctors were not bad people. I suspected some might enjoy the power they wield over patients, and were quick to make other people's decisions for them. However, there had to be some other explanation for the strange things which were happening to us.

The actions of psychologists were not difficult to understand. Their commitment to psychotherapy was a religious faith. Medical doctors, ones who were not particularly enthusiastic about psychiatry, were harder to account for. I was never able to think of but one explanation: They were all involved in research—some secret research no one would discuss with us. Believing we were victims of something impersonal, like a research project, diffused some of my resentment. Feeling oneself to be the victim of a specific tormentor, such as a "rejecting parent". (as psychotherapy often encourages) would have felt worse.

It did seem therapists everywhere were actively recruiting "disturbed" and autistic children as patients. Announcements in newspapers spoke of "spectacular results". The "spectacular results" were rarely spelled out. Cooperation among researchers might explain Colonel Mann's belief that psychiatry had some claim upon Tony which other doctors would respect. Certainly everywhere we turned we encountered coercion to return to psychotherapy. The year Tony was six he attended public school kindergarten. Both the teacher and the school psychologist tried to persuade us to return to the Child Guidance Clinic.

"School is no substitute for treatment," they would warn. I avoided them both as much as possible.

Tony flunked kindergarten. By the next year he was obviously not mature enough for first grade. Marin County had excellent classes for retarded children, and unbeknownst to us, they even conducted a special class for autistic children. We were not told of the class for autistic children, and Tony was not allowed in in classes for the retarded. The school psychologist claimed it was illegal for autistic children to attend special-education classes. For a while I was filled with anger toward the entire California legislature.

Then, common sense told me such a law, if it even existed, could only have been passed at the instigation of scientists concerned with research. What possible motive could legislators have for maliciously denying services to autistic children? There *were* schools Tony could have attended. The cost of schools for "disturbed" children was not in money; parents were required to submit to psychiatric treatment. Some parents were able to pretend to participate in therapy in return for a school for their autistic child. However, Ike and I now understood the purpose of the therapy, and didn't feel capable of such hypocrisy. Tony stayed home for the next three years. One day I read in the newspaper of a proposed meeting in San Francisco for parents of disturbed children.

"Let's go," I said to Ike, "and find out if those children resemble Tony."

"We don't want to become involved with more psychiatrists," Ike cautioned.

"I won't argue," I promised. "I won't say a word. We'll just sit and listen."

Ike agreed, and we looked for a baby sitter. We rarely went anywhere without the children during those years. Tony was becoming difficult to handle, but a good friend agreed to stay with the children. Ike and I found the address, a residence. There didn't seem to be other cars parked in front. We were probably early. The president of the organization, who was the father of a disturbed child, answered the door. Ike and I discussed our children with him and his wife while awaiting other parents. A psychiatrist and a social worker arrived, both young and pleasant. We tried to make small talk. After a while it became apparent Ike and I were going to be the only parents to show up for this meeting, making it awkward to sit and listen.

"We may as well begin," the psychiatrist finally said. He explained that the organization conducted a school for disturbed children. They had six students, and psychiatric treatment for the parents was a basic part of their program. Ike and I were silent.

"We really called this meeting in the hope of doing something nice for the parents of our disturbed children," the pretty young social worker said. "Perhaps you have suggestions?" Ike and I, sitting together on the couch, drew uneasily together, and she continued. "Maybe we could form a little study group to discuss such things as: When Daddy comes home from work tired, and the roast is burned, what Daddy says, and how we react?"

I had promised not to argue but I cringed.

"I bought my wife a meat thermometer," Ike said. "There is no excuse for burned roasts in our house." It was a flippant comment, but I was grateful to Ike for it.

"I sure prefer a meat thermometer to any little study group," I said.

"Well, I suppose a meat thermometer might be one solution,." the social worker agreed vaguely.

I turned to the psychiatrist and asked what happened to disturbed children when they grew up. He said he didn't know, but thought some grew up to be eccentric. I'd always thought of eccentricities as charming quirks of character, signs of individuality, but apparently the psychiatrist regarded them as defects, similar to neuroses.

I tried to tactfully explain my distaste for psychiatry to the likable young doctor, and he seemed to acknowledge dislike of therapy was within our right. Ike and I got up to leave, promising to "keep in touch", think about enrolling Tony in their school.

"There are more than one kind of psychiatrist," the doctor explained as though wanting to explain his positiion. "One kind treats patients; others conduct research."

I should have insisted he explain further, but my mind was in slow motion again. I still had not mastered the ability to pin down doctors. I assumed research would soon reveal the truth about disturbed children, and I was willing to wait.

I never expected to wait the rest of my life.

One day a social worker knocked at our door and claimed she'd been hired by the county to go from house to house searching for disturbed children not in school. She urged me to resume therapy and enroll Tony in a school for disturbed children. A new school for disturbed children was announced in the local paper. Psychiatric treatment for the family was a condition of admission. The school never opened, for they were unable to recruit students. A story about an autistic child was shown on television. The mother didn't like psychiatric treatment any more than I had. In the story, she finally agreed to submit to psychotherapy in return for her child's admission to a special school. She agreed that anything she said during therapy might be used in research. Whoever was promoting research and psychiatric treatment for parents of such children seemed to have unlimited power and resources. I felt alone and helpless.

I kept in touch with the mother whose little boy, Eric, had been diagnosed minimal brain damaged and autistic at the birth defects clinic. She introduced me to an organization for parents of neurologically handicapped children. Many of these parents had also rebelled against psychiatry, but their children took various drugs, such as tranquilizers or antidepressants. The children attended a special nursery school, which charged the parents a modest fee and was said to be partially funded by the county. I applied for Tony's admission.

Again, reports were requested from the Child Guidance Clinic, the birth defects clinic and all doctors who had ever seen Tony. After months of waiting, someone finally called from the school to say they had made a decision about Tony. When I arrived for my appointment, I was surprised to meet the same psychiatric social worker who had interviewed Ike and me at the birth defects clinic two years earlier, the nice lady with whom we had been so trustingly frank. Now she seemed to hold some position with this nursery school and stated Tony would not be allowed to attend unless he were under the care of a psychiatrist.

"The other children aren't under the care of psychiatrists," I protested, fighting back tears of disappointment and frustration.

"Your child is disturbed." She seemed to notice my shocked disbelief. "That was the opinion of the pediatrician in charge of the birth defects clinic," she added sternly.

I remembered that the pediatrician told us neurologists called such children brain damaged, and psychiatrists called them disturbed. Nevertheless, how could I argue with the social worker, part of the all-powerful medical profession, and apparently holding some official position in more than one organization concerned with atypical children?

"Your child needs help," she said. "You can't allow him to stay home and vegetate."

Unable to control them any longer, I left in tears. She wouldn't call it vegetating if she had to keep up with Tony for one day, I thought bitterly. Since he stopped attending school Tony devoted himself full time to mischief, an activity for which he had talent. Many toddlers do things Tony did, but Tony was a terrible-two-year-old for more than ten years. He was a physically capable terrible-two-year-old with a formidable imagination. He appeared impressed (although sometimes a little puzzled) when we scolded him, but every day he was able to think of some startling new mischief. He sprinkled scouring powder on the rug; poured pepper in the stew; dismantled the sewing machine and all the clocks; filled the sugar canister with water; sent an old tire crashing down the hill through a window; threw rocks at the neighbors, and laughed gleefully when they scolded him; swung from telephone wires, which he could reach from the top of a fence; poured pancake syrup in the piano; poured bleach in the washing machine onto colored clothes; put dirt in his father's shaving mug; and smashed anything breakable. I once found him slinging coke bottles from an upstairs porch onto the concrete walk below, apparently because he loved the sound of splintering glass. He painted pictures on the windows with catsup and mayonnaise. In those days Tony's pictures, though not otherwise remarkable, included proper use of perspective. It was a skill no one taught him and one he later lost. Once, he poured salad oil all over the kitchen floor. Then, with the notion maybe he should clean this up, he added a bottle of dish soap and mixed them together with a mop. My feet flew out from under me when I entered the kitchen. I tried to crawl back out of the room, but the floor was too slippery for crawling. I floundered for several minutes before reaching the door.

A neighbor was frightened late one night when hearing noises outside her third-floor, bedroom window. She watched in alarm as the window opened. Then, a small, bare foot appeared over the sill. Tony crawled in the window, laughed, and ran down the stairs and out the door. Getting out of bed, he had climbed over the roof and along a narrow ledge to reach her window.

Tony liked heights and watched television from the top of our big old upright piano. He never fell or injured himself. He demolished two beds by playfully jumping on them. He slammed his bedroom door so hard it split in half. Exuberance, inquisitiveness and love of teasing were usually behind Tony's destructiveness. He did love to tease. He also had a temper though, and sometimes acted like a "disturbed" child, tearing up books and ripping his curtains or clothes to shreds, for instance.

Tony's emotions were exaggerated. When frightened, he was more terrified than other children. When angry he was more furious; when busy, he was quiet and intent. And when Tony was happy, he was exuberantly joyful. For a while, he would leap, squealing with laughter, from the top of the refrigerator onto the shoulders of whoever passed through the kitchen.

Tony's senses were acute. If someone quietly mentioned the word doctor during conversation, Tony could hear from another part of the house, and would yell, "No doctor!" He could find Christmas fruit or chocolate hidden in the back of a closet by his sense of smell. Refusal, or inability, to make eye contact is sometimes listed as a characteristic of autism. Tony's gaze, however, was strikingly direct.

He had an uncanny ability to remember directions. We once went to Disneyland, having been there five years earlier, and Tony pointed out street directions to us. He insisted things be done in certain ways. He kept rugs perfectly straight. He saw that all cupboard and closet doors were closed. During a trip to the hospital, I was amazed at the number of drawers doctors carelessly left open. Tony was busy darting in and out of offices, startling doctors, nurses and patients, trying to close them. His objection to open drawers wasn't because he was neat. Tony's table manners were atrocious. Most of his idiosyncrasies disappeared after a while, to be replaced by new ones.

At seven or eight Tony was a beautiful child. He had the lovely, pink-cheeked complexion of a baby. A radiant smile lit up his face, and his big blue eyes sparkled with fun and mischief. Strangers rarely suspected the mental development of such a busy, curious, alert looking child could be retarded. His behavior was difficult to explain. I took him to the playground but he got along badly with other children. If they so much as touched him, he might lose his temper and throw sand at them. Once, he playfully pushed over a baby, making her cry.

"Why you little devil," the mother exclaimed. She jumped up to chase Tony, who laughed and ran.

"I'm sorry," I apologized, my face burning with humiliation. "My little boy doesn't understand."

"I'll bet he'd understand my shoe on his behind if I could catch him," she muttered, unconvinced anything was wrong with Tony other than deviltry.

When I took him with me to visit anyone, he would do something outrageous. For instance I had hardly settled myself in a friend's living room with a cup of tea, when a dripping cat raced by us. Tony had thrown it in the swimming pool. Then her electricity went off. Later she discovered Tony had disconnected the fuse boxes. Staying home with him seemed easiest. Life wasn't simple. We were too busy to wonder if we were "happy". Ike and I were struggling financially, as well as trying to cope with Tony. Today I remember with pleasure those years when the children were small. (Except for my encounters with doctors, whom I avoided when possible.) Fishing was Ike's recreation, and Tony did well on camping trips. We enjoyed Little League games, Blue Birds, Cub Scouts, the children's dance and music recitals, school performances, Sunday picnics and trips to the zoo and museums. At times I felt desperate, but I tried not to think about Tony's future. I reminded myself the possessions Tony destroyed were expendable. By disciplining myself not to care what strangers thought, I managed to endure Tony's mischief and destructiveness with a show of serenity. I felt I had no choice, remembering the long list of psychologists eager to offer me a couch if I wanted to complain.

We finally persuaded Army dentists to fix Tony's teeth. He had to be hospitalized and given a general anesthetic. The mysterious pains in his ears, nose, teeth or head continued. Occasionally they were in his arms or legs. Tony was unusually sensitive to pain, and maybe these were sensations most people could ignore. He was ingenious at thinking of remedies, and rubbed mashed potatoes, toothpaste, pancake syrup or mayonnaise on his hurt— usually in his hair. Sometimes when he got one of these mysterious pains he would scream and slap the painful spot, or knock his head against the wall. He was careful to pick a wall where he wouldn't injure himself, such as the soft, crumbly plaster of our old house. Tony was knocking huge holes in every room, and our house looked as though an earthquake had struck. Being unable to do anything for our little boy was heartbreaking. I occasionally tried to find medical treatment for him, but doctors I consulted only suggested, helplessly, we return to the psychiatric clinic.

Once at a neurology clinic I was surprised to learn one of the neurologists was also a psychiatrist.

"I understand neurologists consider children like Tony brain damaged, and psychiatrists believe they are suffering from maternal rejection. Which theory do *you* favor?" I asked.

"I'm not partial to either theory, but there is one matter on which we all agree: These children don't stand a chance without some treatment, either psychotherapy or some type of drug therapy," he warned.

The neurologists prescribed a tranquilizer. I gave it to Tony for a couple of weeks without effect. His head banging continued off and on for several years.

Tony was nine and hadn't attended school for two years, when the school psychologist contacted me and assigned Tony a home teacher. Tony had no understanding of reading and writing, and didn't talk as well as the average four-year-old. However I was grateful for someone to pay attention to him a few hours a week.

At Tony's end-of-the-term school conference, the school psychologist tried to persuade me to try a drug therapy, offering a choice of several tranquilizers and antidepressants.

I'd read school psychologists all over the country were prescribing drugs for hyperactive children. I knew the effectiveness of these drugs had not been demonstrated. No doctor had made a serious effort to find out what was with Tony, and I didn't fancy giving him drugs on such an experimental basis.

"Drugs might relax Tony and allow him to learn more," the psychologist argued.

I've already tried a tranquilizer and an antidepressant. Neither had much effect."

"Are you afraid of side effects?"

"Oh I suppose there are no grossly harmful side effects, but all drugs have some. I don't want to give a drug to Tony without evidence it might help."

The psychologist argued a few more minutes, finally lapsing into silence.

"I hear you won't be with our school district next year," I commented to change the subject.

"That's right," he answered absently. "I'm going into private practice. My only connection with the school district now is a research project on which I'm still working."

I approved of research, and might have cooperated if anyone had been honest with us. I resented my local school district trying to pressure me into unproven treatments, feeling I should be offered more choice about participating in medical experiments. A few years later a law was passed requiring parents' informed consent before involving children in research. But in 1966 social scientists were confident that their wondrous 20th century technology could eventually remake humanity to conform to their scientific view of how people should be. Most professionals seemed to assume such a goal justified any tactic.

Chapter 14

Is it the patient or the therapist who benefits?

A clinic at San Francisco State College, funded by the State Department of Education, was frankly and openly involved in research. Many of my friends' neurologically handicapped children had been diagnosed there. The doctors were reputedly not psychiatrically oriented. The clinic was headed by a neurologist, and they looked for physical causes of abnormal development. I requested an evaluation for Tony. The waiting list was long, and Tony was nearly ten when we went for his examination. A social worker interviewed me.

"What did the Child Guidance Clinic diagnose your son?" he asked when I explained Tony had been treated there for two years.

"No one ever told us," I answered.

"Do you mean six years after first taking your little boy to a doctor, you still don't know his diagnosis?"

I shook my head, grateful someone finally agreed our experience seemed appalling.

"When we finish examining your child, you and your husband will meet with all the specialists examining Tony. Each will report their findings," he said. "We'll answer all your questions and give you a diagnosis."

His sincerity and concern seemed obvious. Had I finally found doctors I could trust? My naturally optimistic nature surged, and I forgot the bewilderment and heart-break I'd felt after each doctor had been devious. This time was going to be different.

Doctors, speech and hearing specialists, teachers and psychologists examined Tony for four days. I watched Tony take some tests. He could work jigsaw puzzles and fit things together. Tony completed a test labeled "space relations" in an instant, even before the tester told him what to do. He had no comprehension of tests requiring him to distinguish articles found in hardware stores from those found in clothing stores.

The physical examination was not extensive. Doctors still lacked technology to reveal much of what went on in the brain. However, Tony was examined by the neurologist. In order to determine dominance, the neurologist suggested Tony kick him. Tony hauled off and delivered a whack on his shin with his right foot. The neurologist winced, probably not expecting such enthusiasm. Tony was left-handed, and had mixed dominance.

We drove to the clinic on the fifth day. On the way I stopped by the Child Guidance Clinic at the Presidio to pick up Tony's records, which had been requested but never sent. Then I stopped the car in Golden Gate Park. Prying the staples out of the folder, I spent a few minutes reading Tony's medical records. I read the letter from the doctor at the Child Guidance Clinic stating their treatment had been curing Tony of his illness, but he regressed whenever he was returned to the family situation, and "when this became apparent to the mother she suddenly withdrew the child from treatment." I wondered if I should remove the letter from Tony's file. No, I decided. It was a ridiculous allegation to make against any Mother, and only revealed the psychologists' lack of objectivity. The social worker's assurances had been emphatic. All these specialists and scientists associated with a college surely wouldn't have wasted four and a half days examining Tony if they were going to take the word of some silly Army psychologists who saw him four years ago.

"Let's go! Let's go!" Tony urged, eager to get to the clinic. He was enjoying the various tests and examinations. I closed the file and drove on for the final day of his evaluation.

Before our concluding conference that morning, I had an appointment with a psychiatrist. The psychiatrist hadn't appeared to be an important member of the examining team. This was the first day he'd been at the clinic. The appointment was scheduled for only fifteen minutes, probably an unimportant, routine interview. The psychiatrist, a small, dark haired man, seemed to lack enthusiasm for his job. His woeful brown eyes suggested a permanent expression of melancholy.

"I see from Tony's records a child guidance clinic has already diagnosed him," he said.

"Tony was seen there," I answered, "but they never told us their diagnosis."

"Autistic is what they say here in their report."

"I remember a psychologist mentioning that term but I don't know what it means."

"Would you consider taking Tony to Langly Porter Psychiatric Clinic?" he asked after a moment of gloomy silence.

I knew people whose children were treated at Langly Porter. The treatment was psychotherapy.

"No. I'm sorry. I don't believe in that type of treatment."

The psychiatrist frowned.

"I don't really believe in psychotherapy as a treatment for any illness," I added as diffidently as I could. I suspected psychiatrists might be annoyed by a suggestion that psychotherapy couldn't cure anything. Nevertheless, I had read a growing number of doctors were convinced mental illness had physical causes. Surely I was also entitled to such a view.

The psychiatrist sat staring despondently at the floor. He waved his hand, indicating I could leave. I returned to the waiting room. In a few minutes the social worker sent for me, the man who had promised all our questions would be answered today.

"So far as you are concerned this is the first time anyone has actually examined Tony, isn't it?"

I'd already told him that. He seemed agitated. Were he and the psychiatrist having some disagreement about Tony?

"Yes, this is the first time anyone has given him a physical examination," I said.

He didn't seem to want anything else from me. I returned uneasily to the waiting room. Had something gone wrong? Surely after all these years we couldn't still "belong" to the psychiatrists.

The psychiatrist sent for me again.

"Have you ever noticed Tony sit and rock back and forth and stare into space, unaware of his surroundings?" he asked.

"No, the most abnormal appearing thing Tony does is demand we repeat things."

"He makes you repeat words or phrases with the same tone of voice?"

"Yes. And sometimes if we touch him, he insists we touch him again in the same spot."

Still looking glum, the psychiatrist dismissed me again. I returned to the waiting room. All these professionals had seemed straight forward and candid all week. Now, with the arrival of the psychiatrist, things were getting strange. *Oh please don't let this evaluation turn into another disaster!*

I felt too nervous to sit and talk to the other mothers in the waiting room. Their children only had problems in school, and doctors usually diagnosed them as having a learning disability. I went out to pace up and down the hall. As I passed the social worker's office, he stuck his head out, furtively motioned me in and closed the door. He didn't ask me to sit down.

"You are going to listen to our diagnosis today—pardon me, I mean our *opinion*—and then do what you think is best for Tony, aren't you?" he asked. He stood uneasy by door the door waiting for my answer.

"That's what I've always done."

"Yes," he agreed distractedly, as he cautiously opened the door for me to leave. As the door closed behind me, any hopes I had been clinging to plummeted. This examination was turning out to be as bewildering as the others. They were apparently planning to tell us something with which the social worker disagreed. Most medical doctors who felt compelled to be devious during those years appeared uncomfortable at being less than candid. On the other hand, psychologists rarely appeared embarrassed when trying to maneuver patients, considering manipulation of people to be one of their skills. This social worker was the exception, and I remember with gratitude he at least seemed to feel badly about whatever they were doing.

I returned and sat woodenly in the waiting room, with growing dread and apprehension. By the time Ike arrived and we went in for our conference, my insides felt like they were made of lead. The somber looks on the faces of the three doctors, who were seated behind a long table on a raised platform, confirmed my dread. The dozen or so people who had examined Tony during the week were not there, as the social worker had promised. Only the psychiatrist, the social worker and the neurologist in charge of the clinic looked down upon us from behind the table. Ike and I sat down in the front row of empty chairs. The silence felt oppressive. The psychiatrist began to speak in a bleak tone.

"We're sorry to tell you your child is severely retarded, not educable…" He dropped Tony's records on the table in a gesture of hopelessness. "Eventual institutionalization is his only prospect. He's not autistic, as I first thought…" He kept hesitating as though expecting us to protest. If he thought Tony was autistic an hour ago, how could he now be so certain of another diagnosis without examining Tony? "Or if he is emotionally disturbed," the psychiatrist continued despondently, "the condition has already gone so long without treatment the illness is probably irreversible..."

I guess I've always suspected retardation," Ike said.

I sat there, trying not to feel anything. I was determined not to fall apart, struggling not to cry. I couldn't think of a question to ask. My mind was paralyzed again.

"We believe public institutions are better than private ones," the neurologist continued. "You people are not as young as you might be. There are advantages to making your child a ward of the state."

I should think of some question to ask.

The doctors were watching us silently. Apparently our conference was over.

"It's his central nervous system," the neurologist said as we got up to leave. "There are drugs he can be given: Dexadrine, librium, Valium, Ritalin."

"Those drugs don't cure retardation," I heard myself protest.

Ike and I left. The social worker had remained silent throughout the conference.

The thought of Tony in an institution devastated me. He loved to eat. Sometimes he could consume a pound of hot dogs at one meal. Pizza and spaghetti were other favorites, and he would devour leftovers the next morning for breakfast. And cookies—no one in a public institution would bake cookies for Tony. One night recently he had called from his bedroom,

"Mommy, bwing you toof pick!"

Tony confused pronouns. Fortunately, it isn't necessary to clarify pronouns for normal children. Anyone who attempts to explain "you" really means "me", and "I" means "you", will discover how entangled such explanations become, deteriorating into something like a "who's-on-first routine". Gestures only add confusion.

I got out of bed and took Tony a toothpick. But Tony didn't want it for his teeth. He was lying in bed with a dish of olives on his chest and a self-satisfied sparkle in his eyes. He wanted the toothpick with which to eat his olives. The rest of the family came in and laughed at him. Tony laughed too.

In spite of the problems he caused, we all enjoyed Tony. The children's friends thought Tony was "neat". He was like a three year old, a delightful, independent, imaginative, mischievous little three year old. I remembered how quiet and lonely the house had seemed while Tony was in the hospital having his teeth fixed. Tony's independence didn't mean he didn't love us. He would be frightened and unhappy in an institution among strangers.

No one could force us to put Tony in an institution, I finally reminded myself. Perhaps we should have sued someone. However our generation did not expect financial compensation for every personal misfortune, and in those days even lawyers probably agreed pursuit of scientific research justified any means. I felt such resentment I was unable to discuss doctors without bursting into tears. We had neither energy nor money to waste on lawsuits

I never saw the results of any research that might have involved Tony. However I suspected what social scientists might do with evidence that did not confirm their expectations: declare the experiment a failure and bury the results.

I once found an obscure research project in an old psychology book. In 1935, a massive effort was undertaken to prove crime can be prevented. It was called the Cambridge-Sommerville Youth Study. Boys who had been in trouble, and were considered pre-delinquent, were referred to the project by welfare agencies, police, churches and schools. To avoid stigmatizing the group, an equal number of normal boys were included. The boys, an average age of nine, were divided into pairs. Each pair was equated as nearly as possible as to health, intelligence, emotional adjustment, economic class, home atmosphere, neighborhood and delinquency prognosis. Thus the project started with 325 matched sets. The flip of a coin determined which boy of each pair would be treated, and which would go into the control group. The families of those in the control group were interviewed, but otherwise left to the resources of the community. The boys in the treatment group received attention from doctors, psychologists, psychiatrists, special tutors, counselors, and constant guidance from their own personal social worker.

Treatment ended in 1945 when the boys were in their middle teens. Twenty and thirty-year, follow up studies indicate the treated boys fared slightly worse than those who were left alone. The treated group committed more and worse crimes, were more often alcoholic, had more mental illness and were more dissatisfied with their lives.

If scientific tests could be devised which determined whether psychotherapy actually helps or hurts people, I wonder what the result would be? I realize some people who undergo therapy enjoy the attention, but could such dependence upon a therapist merely further postpone a patient's ability to make independent decisions?

CHAPTER 15

Would perfection be a handicap?

The most important aspects of our humanity seem beyond the scope of science, for they cannot be measured—courage, compassion integrity, tenacity, patience, generosity and honor, as well as their opposites. (What would be the meaning of honor without the existence of dishonor?) Such qualities used to be attributed to a soul, but that term has been ridiculed during this age of scientific materialism. Many materialists have argued such character traits are not part of a person at birth, but are learned, taught by parents and society. Maybe some children are that malleable, but I knew my children were each born a complete person, an individual with their own character, personality and indomitable soul, and their own talents, wants, abilities, defects and limitations.

I always had the feeling Tony, if he weren't retarded, might have resembled his older brother. Our only child to suffer serious illness, Guy was born with pyloric stenosis, an obstruction between the stomach and the intestines. Ike and I were terrified when our firstborn had to undergo surgery at the age of two weeks, but he quickly recovered, reinforcing our faith in the magical powers of medical science. He didn't talk until three, and was slow to learn to play with other children and to acquire social skills. Before he started kindergarten, I attempted to teach him a little about numbers and the alphabet. He tried, but obviously wasn't yet capable of such comprehension. By the first grade he seemed able to learn at the rate of other children. While he didn't lack all ability to imitate people, as Tony did, he had less of that talent than most children had. A quiet little boy when not asking questions, he was inclined to daydreaming and absent-mindedness, sometimes forgetting where he was going on the way to school. He liked school well enough, but was preoccupied with the significance of prehistoric men, molecules and infinity. Once when he was six, he had a disagreement with a neighbor boy and wrote him an angry letter:

> *Dear Elmer,*
> *You are a pithecanthropus.*
> *Love,*
> *Guy*

"I'll bet that'll make him mad," Guy said, "'Cause he won't know what it means."

Nothing upset Guy more than not understanding the meaning of something. Independent like Tony, he announced he was now too old for all that hugging-and-kissing stuff. I had to admit I understood. I also felt dismayed by friends or acquaintances who greet me by grabbing hold of me and made smacking noises near my ear. A wet kiss would be even worse. Guy considered fairy tales and children's fiction a hoax, and preferred to read science books. When I first took Tony to the pediatrician, and got the feeling doctors suspected high intelligence, Guy was in the third grade. He finished reading his first set of children's encyclopedias and requested a more advanced set. Fearing some ticklish problem, such as whether my child should skip a grade in school, I avoided his teacher. To my chagrin, Guy's school problems turned out to be quite different. He had to struggle to learn some things other children pick up effortlessly. He began coming home from school crying, not sure himself why he was unhappy. Our attempts to discover the cause of his misery always ended in a discussion of arithmetic.

"Arithmetic wouldn't be so bad if sometimes four and four could be seven and sometimes it could be nine. But it's always eight." he protested. "And the next day it's still eight. I hate it!"

"But Honey, you had no trouble with arithmetic in the first and second grades," I said.

"I know. I did it on my fingers. This year I don't have enough fingers."

His mysterious unhappiness vanished the moment school was out for the summer. Guy admired his fourth-grade teacher, a man, and enjoyed school again. However Guy perplexed his teacher. At our school conference he said,

"This kid has me baffled. He's smart, attentive and interested—but he doesn't do especially well. He's peculiar. Well, I don't actually mean peculiar," the teacher apologized, as he noticed me cringe at his reference to the family abnormality. "He's a terrific little boy, but he's...well...I don't know...peculiar."

The school provided funds for a special project for the "more able learners" of the class. They made rockets. The teacher invited Guy to participate even though he obviously wasn't a "more able learner". Guy enjoyed the rocket project, but it didn't turn him into a "more able learner". The teacher also asked the class to write a composition describing a personal problem, and what the student had done to solve it. Guy's compositions were always concise, and this one consisted of one sentence:

"My personal problems are my own personal business."

Privately, I was proud of Guy's "essay". Maybe he'd not be inclined to blame his problems on someone else when he grew up.

Guy's fourth-grade teacher was concerned his grades might not be good enough for college, but I never worried. Although not articulate, he was consumed by curiosity.

"I think it was a big 'splosion, myself," he might say.

"What was a big explosion?"

"The beginning of the universe. Cause there sure had to be a lot of heat to make all that 'tomic energy," he would decide.

"Well I guess there are two theories—"

"It's probably 'herited, but not by just one gene."

"What's inherited?"

"Schizophrenia. Maybe I'll do a project about that for the science fair this year."

I pictured how impressed the teachers might be by Guy's views on the cause of schizophrenia. (Actually, they have proven to be more valid than the fanciful speculations about damaged psyches in which most psychiatrists were indulging at that time.)

"I know what all the symbols stand for, but I wonder what the whole thing really means?"

"What symbols?"

"E equals m,c squared. You know, Mommy, yesterday the teacher said light always travels in a straight line. I raised my hand 'cause I wanted to ask about Einstein saying it travels in a curve. The bell rang and I didn't get a chance, though."

Too bad the bell rang just then. It might have been interesting to know how fourth-grade teachers answer such a question.

Guy used to insist he was incapable of memorizing anything. The Boy Scout oath was his first success and required weeks of effort. He is grown now and has apparently acquired an adequate memory. Married to a Russian, he has learned to speak that language so fluently they speak it at home. He also speaks Spanish.

Guy's differences were never extreme enough for anyone to call him "withdrawn". Now an absent-minded professor, and an accomplished musician, he gets along with people because he's unselfish, kind and considerate. He has little talent for small talk. His goals and aspirations are rarely typical. Like the rest of the family, he is concerned with philosophical questions and committed to pondering the difference between right and wrong. Happily married, he is beloved by his family, and well liked by his students and colleagues. Many people find his eccentricities charming.

When Guy was ten, he once declared,

"Even if I can't learn the multiplication tables, I'm still glad I'm me!"

While I never succeeded in eradicating regret of Tony's retardation, I always hoped none of my children, including Tony, would waste energy deploring their own unique natures.

From birth, our daughter's personality differed from that of her brothers. A demonstratively affectionate, imaginative, outgoing child, she talked early. Once when she was two, Guy came to complain Sherry wasn't doing her share of picking up toys in their room. I heard him go back and announce to his baby sister,

"Mommy says if I do all the work, I'll get all the credit."

"Cwedit-Hmph!," scoffed Sherry, lounging lazily on her bed, sucking her thumb. "What's cwedit? What can you do wif it? Is it good to eat? Can you put it up on the dwesser and look at it?"

Sherry did not turn out to be the realist these precocious comments might have indicated. She loved fairy tales and was people oriented. When she began kindergarten she rushed home every day, eager to share her experiences. One day she breathlessly related,

"Today, Mommy, the teacher told about a blinkin. This blinkin just roamed through the woods all day, looking for books, 'cause it wanted to read. And when it grew up, Mommy, it became the United States of America! Or maybe a man. I'm not sure which. Anyway, there's another man. I think his name is George. And they both have birthdays this month."

Her entertaining remarks were often based on willingness to repeat something she didn't understand. Once when Sherry was playing house, Guy asked how many children she planned to have when she grew up.

"Three," she answered, "a boy, a girl and one like Tony just for fun."

Some people have reported feeling embarrassed about a retarded sibling when young. I don't think Guy and Sherry were ever ashamed of Tony. He was cute and funny. The things he did were startlingly unexpected. In any case, many children learn to cope with such problems without emotional damage. If Tony had been less attractive, I hope my children would have also profited from dealing with such painful feelings at a young age.

Sherry showed immaturity by reversing letters in the second grade, but her school problems were never serious. She is now a nurse and mother. Not only is she intuitive and sensitive to people, she has the ability to remain cool during emergencies. (Her brothers and I are disasters when the panic button is pushed.) When she was a child she was walking by a parked car that began to roll. Although she didn't know how to drive, she opened the door and put her hand on the brake until an adult came to the rescue. Like the rest of the family, Sherry is concerned with metaphysical questions, forms her own opinions, and is not bothered if her beliefs are unconventional. She is involved in holistic medicine. However I think Sherry learned to reach her own conclusions after becoming an adult. Her brothers seemed to lack much of the normal childhood ability to absorb other people's beliefs and attitudes.

Sherry's son, Colin, possesses that mysterious ability to pick up appropriate behaviors. Since birth he has understood people, charming anyone who came with ten feet of him. He began trying to organize the diaper set at the playground while still two. He would lie about his age, once telling a four year old he was six.

"I'm lots bigger than you," scoffed the four year old.

Colin thought a few seconds, and then declared indifferently, "Ha. Ha. Ha." It was sophisticated repartee for a two year old.

After his first week of kindergarten, he confided to his mother, "I have a problem. I have a tendency to be just a little bit bossy." (Obviously a teacher's criticism.)

He wanted to play the violin, but when the music class was offered at his school, Colin was the only five year old expressing an interest. In an effort to organize such a class, he talked three of his classmates into studying the violin. (Anyone who can persuade a bunch of five year olds to take up the violin is surely more of a leader than some Cub Scout den mother.)

      *   *   *

A couple of years ago, I attended the christening of a grandchild, Guy's firstborn daughter.

"You came all the way from California for the christening," exclaimed the Russian priest.

Although I had only learned of the event the night before upon my arrival in Pennsylvania, I smiled in demure acknowledgment of his praise. Three flags decorated the alter: the flag of Pennsylvania, the American flag, and the flag of the Czar. The priest, six and a half feet and more than two hundred pounds, dominated the tiny Russian Orthodox Church. He wore colorful embroidered robes over embroidered velvet robes and had a big black beard. There were no chairs in a Russian church; everyone stood. The godmother belonged to another Russian church than the one my daughter-in-law attended. Christening ceremonies of both churches were performed, each seeming endless. The priest and his attendants circled the room, swinging a smoking bronze incense burner and chanting in Russian. Finally they returned to the alter, and the priest began painting crosses on each of the baby's tiny joints with a little watercolor brush dipped in holy water.

"What's he doing?" I whispered to my son.

"He's exorcizing demons and rebellious thoughts," Guy whispered back.

Just one moment, I was tempted to protest, as an indignant grandmother. What was wrong with rebellious thoughts? Even my charming grandson, Colin has a rebellious thought now and then.

The priest had probably been in this country since the Russian revolution, but some of his attitudes had remained Russian. Our society once valued obedience more highly. Wives obeyed husbands, children obeyed parents and teachers, students accepted academic authorities without challenge, people obeyed their rulers and government officials, and no one questioned the established religion. (I had to admit obedience allowed society to function smoothly.)

The priest finished painting crosses on each of Eve's tiny pink toes. Then he picked her up and dunked her three times in the pot of holy water. Eve exploded into a violent bundle of screaming rage.

I relaxed. Any granddaughter of mine would surely always be capable of a few rebellious thoughts.

My Russian granddaughter, Elena, a competent little girl, was nine when she arrived in this country. She ate five pounds of bananas, acquired a Barbie doll and became an instant American. Although quickly won over to the benefits of an affluent society, she still professed an ambition to become a member of the Supreme Soviet when she grew up.

"You have to live in Russia to be a member of the Supreme Soviet," we pointed out.

"Why?" she exclaimed, "I already lived there nine years!" (More than nine years without bananas and Barbie dolls shouldn't be expected of any little girl.) During her first four months in this country, Elena attended school, unable to speak or understand a word. There was no bilingual education for Russian children. Within three years she caught up with her age group in school, and was an American teenager. We were watching ET on Television. When ET became ill, the government scientists burst officiously into the house to take him to their laboratory.

"The government can't walk into someone's house without permission," our little ex-communist exclaimed in almost unaccented English. "Why I'd haul them into court and sue their sox off!"

Bertha Jane, my youngest grandchild, will be the next scientist in the family, Her father reports. Someone recently told her she was pretty.

"Well, I'm probably going to get glasses, braces, curly hair and freckles," she replied, unimpressed.

I'm confident none of my grandchildren will be perfect. That is a fate I wouldn't wish upon any child. I fear perfect children might grow up to be similar, successful, untroubled, perennially-contented, useful citizens— people who could only age, never grow. Psychologists argue the nature-nurture controversy, sometimes announcing, for instance, a trait is sixty percent inherited and forty percent due to environment— free-will being assigned zero percent! (Maybe some of us have more free will than others, and people who don't believe in it don't have much.) My children and grandchildren may have been born with certain strengths and weaknesses, but each of them consists of something more than a collection of atoms interacting according to understandable physical laws and powered by a mechanical device called a brain, which is regarded as something resembling a computer. A materialist might claim that since "free will" can't be measured, it is not real. However my children and grandchildren each have an unmeasurable will of their own, which will determine whatever success or failure they make of their particular talents and deficits.

CHAPTER 16

An inoculation against throwing rocks

The clinic where we were told Tony was hopelessly retarded was part of San Francisco State College, an institution funded by the State Department of Education. Tony, aged ten, now had an official diagnosis of retardation, and I told myself he must surely be eligible for special education classes. I again contacted our school psychologist. Instead of a class for the retarded, Tony was admitted to a class for autistic children, an experimental class using operant conditioning. The children were rewarded with a piece of candy for each desirable response.

"It's illegal to use special-education funds for this class, because the children aren't retarded," the school psychologist sometimes said to the parents conspiratorially, "but we do it anyway."

Most of the children had been in the class for at least a year. They had received many diagnoses, including disturbed, autistic, schizophrenic and neurologically impaired. Their retardation probably had many causes. Unlike Tony, most appeared to have less than perfect nervous systems. It seemed strange the school district had refused to admit Tony to this class while he was diagnosed autistic, but he was now allowed to attend with an official diagnosis of retardation. However, I was grateful that he was finally in school and didn't question anyone.

On the first day Tony sat down in his little chair, stubbornly squeezed his eyes shut and stuck his fingers in his ears.

"Did you ever see such determination not to learn," said the teacher said with a laugh.

Tony's negative attitude was short lived however, and he soon loved school. A bus picked him up every morning and delivered him home in the afternoon. Having a few hours to myself was a luxury, and life became more relaxed for the whole family. Academic subjects were stressed, and the teachers were convinced they were going to cure the children's retardation. They encouraged the parents to think of their children growing up to be doctors and lawyers. Tony was toilet trained by operant conditioning, for us, the most exciting accomplishment of his childhood.

Psychiatry was the first treatment the medical profession proposed for autism. Parents formed organizations and rebelled against psychotherapy. However they wrote in one of their first newsletters, "We aspire to be more than just an anti-psychiatry organization. We must be for something." Parents sometimes made great sacrifices, selling their homes, giving up their jobs and moving across the country in search of some school or therapy for an autistic child. Frightened and desperate, most parents were pathetically eager to see improvement, and most retarded children grew and learned enough for each treatment to be proclaimed a success. Some of these treatments tried over the years included: a variety of drugs, from LSD and anti-psychotic drugs, to vitamins. (Vitamins, though no cure, proved to be the least harmful, but with no pharmaceutical company to promote them, vitamins never attracted a wide following.) Other treatments included "rage therapy" (a psychiatrist screaming at the child), playing with dolphins, hypnosis,

Sensory Integration (playing soft music into the child's ears though ear phones), a multitude of teaching techniques, and "patterning". This last consisted of constant manipulation of the retarded child's arms and legs by the entire family and an army of volunteers. The manipulators, working in relays, could rest, but the retarded child was subjected to the treatment for most of his non-sleeping hours.

"Facilitated communication" was another treatment. A therapist supported the arm of the autistic child, while the child typed profound messages. Some of these children didn't even know the alphabet unless the facilitator was "supporting" their arm. In fact, some of them didn't even look at the keyboard. The facilitator looked.

If these treatments had been offered to us, I would have taken advantage of any which I thought wouldn't harm Tony. I endured therapy for two and a half years so that he could spend an hour a week with a psychologist.

Tony remained in the class for autistic children for three years, and was then transferred to a regular special-education class for "trainable" retarded children. I actually felt more comfortable among parents who were allowed accept their children's handicaps. It was a relief to find parents among whom we could laugh about our children. Parents of "autistic" children were often too frightened to laugh, especially if they felt society expected them to "do something" about their children's problems. I wanted all of my children's childhood to include laughter.

Tony's special-education teachers were skillful and patient, and taught him many things, such as: to distinguish between men and women on restroom doors; not to cross streets at a red light; to make his bed; and to wash his clothes and fold them neatly in his drawer. Special education helps retarded children learn to live in protected environments. It doesn't claim to cure retardation or autism.

Guy and Sherry used to claim with amusement Tony "was only mildly retarded, but severely lazy." After he was taught to make his bed he would sleep on top, instead of between the sheets, so as to avoid that chore. He sometimes seemed to show more intelligence than ability to learn. He never acquired the language, attitudes and appropriate behaviors that even retarded children pick up when young. Such skills allow some "normal" people to get through life without ever "thinking".

He did have talents, however. His curiosity and imagination were unusual for such a retarded child. An invisible playmate, a "big brown pussy-dog named Achi-Cha-Cha", supposedly went roller-skating with him. We allowed Tony to name our new kitten, knowing he would pick something original. He named it Gawgy. Tony's mischief was imaginative and he sometimes told on himself with appealing innocence.

"Tony didn't break your flower," he protested one morning.

I examined the houseplants and found one broken at the stem, but neatly mended with scotch tape.

A stranger, unaware of Tony's retardation, once asked him,

"What do you plan to be when you grow up, young man?"

"Bald on top," Tony replied, leaving his questioner suspecting impertinence.

Although Tony didn't often speak, his occasional startling statements were sometimes delightful. One evening at dinner I was silently nursing a pique because Ike had stopped by the officers club for a few drinks, and Ike was trying to tease me out of my bad mood. Guy and Sherry were eating in silence, electing to remain neutral. Suddenly Tony, who probably hadn't said a word all day, declared,

"Daddy's up to no good!" We all roared with laughter.

The most startling of his behaviors was echolalia, which lasted several months. At about the age of eight and a half, he began echoing with utter lack of comprehension, long sentences he heard on television. He could say "justification for escalating the conflict in Vietnam" without mispronouncing a syllable. Although he learned to state his needs, communication never became easy for Tony. (To this day he prefers not to talk, and must be coaxed into one-word answers to most questions.)

About the age of thirteen Tony began to spin things. He'd twirl a rope or chain, or he'd pick a branch off a tree or bush and walk around shaking it vigorously. He became unable to tolerate scolding. Although I tried to correct him in a calm, quiet voice, he would become upset and demand I repeat whatever said to him. His little quirk seemed harmless enough at first. Then he began insisting we repeat several times. We were unable to prevent irritation from creeping into our voices, which further upset Tony. He also became possessive of me, and would chant "ya-ya-ya" to prevent me from talking to anyone.

Much of the time Tony was happy and playful, but he could also suddenly become enraged and destructive. We were eating in a restaurant one day. How handsome and well-behaved Tony is, I thought, watching him with pride. Then he hit his knee on something under the table. He screamed and began throwing glasses and dishes. I jumped up and tried to hurry him outside past all the silent, stunned people who had stopped eating to gape at his tantrum. He managed to grab one more glass from a table we passed and smash it on the floor.

He came home from school angry and kicked a dent in the side of the school bus. He wasn't allowed back to school for a week. Tony seemed indifferent to his suspension, but I lived in terror that the teachers might decide they couldn't handle him. The first day he was allowed to return to class, he kicked a window out of the bus. I remembered the years when Tony hadn't attended school, and lived in dread that we might be forced to return to that life.

Tony's insistence we repeat things became more difficult to cope with. I tried to joke about it. I threatened him. I tried to bribe him. I laughed. I yelled at him. I cried. I tried to distract him. I spanked him. Finally I announced we were going to refuse to repeat. The family was skeptical, knowing Tony's determination. That evening I was running Tony's bath, and he started to get into the tub.

I said, "No, it's not ready yet."

"Say no it's not ready yet," Tony demanded.

"No, Tony, I'm not going to repeat it."

"Say no it's not ready yet!" he screamed.

I forced myself to remain silent.

He ran out on to the front porch without any clothes on and screamed, "Say no it's not ready yet. Say no it's not ready yet."

I made him get dressed, and he went out in the back yard and screamed and kicked the house and threatened to break windows. I kept a serene expression frozen upon my face, and for some reason Tony didn't carry out his threats. Later I was cooking chicken. Tony came in and tried to take a drumstick.

I said, "No, It's not ready y—" *Oh damn*, I thought, biting off the words. Now he would start all over again.

"Say no it's not ready yet," Tony demanded.

I gritted my teeth and remained silent. Tony finally went off and tried to trick his brother and sister to say the desired words.

We didn't cure Tony of making us repeat things, but he relented a little. Everyone in our special-education department made heroic efforts to solve the problems of each retarded child, and the teachers decided some older, bossy boys on Tony's bus might be upsetting him. They assigned him to transportation with quieter children, and Tony stopped trying to demolish the bus. However if we sometimes thought we'd found reasons for Tony's rages, at other times no one could fathom their cause.

"Tell me how much is four and four or I'll tickle you," Guy would say. This was Tony's favorite game and his face would light up with delight.

"Six!" he would declare impishly, deliberately giving the wrong answer with that crooked little grin and mischievous glimmer in his eyes. When he'd had enough tickling he would squeal, "Four and four is eight."

However, without warning Tony's games and laughter could turn into a nightmare. One evening Guy accidentally bumped into him, making him angry. Tony grabbed a plate from the table and ran out of the house, slamming the door and cracking the glass. He smashed the plate on the concrete walk and threw an old piece of iron crashing through a window. Although splintered glass lay everywhere, as usual,

Tony hadn't cut himself. I got him and took him into his room, removed his shirt and made him get into bed. (Tony ripped up several shirts a week, and I bought them in thrift shops.) Guy and Sherry were trying to help me restrain him. He managed to break loose and kick a hole in the wall.

"The things he does look—well—almost psychotic," Guy said in a frightened voice.

I felt frightened too.

"Tony need spanking?" Tony taunted. We did nothing, and he continued, "Go tell Daddy Tony broke a wall."

Ike appeared. Tony grabbed the curtain, yanking the curtain rod out of the wall. Ike pulled down Tony's pants and spanked him.

"That's what he wants," I said. "It only makes him worse."

"I know," Ike said, "but I'm only human."

Tony picked up a chair and tried to hurl it through a window. We wrested it from him. He caught Sherry's long hair and pulled. We forced him back onto the bed.

"We're not going to be able to handle him much longer," Ike warned. "He's getting bigger and stronger every day. Something has to be done."

None of us ever came out and spoke of putting Tony in an institution, but the prospect lurked in all our minds. I felt sick with fear. Strangers would be less able to handle him than we were. People working in institutions wouldn't love Tony. They would only lock him up. Sherry began to cry.

"There's no point in talking about if we can handle Tony," Guy said. "We have to do it!"

I felt grateful for his support.

"If only we had a way to punish him," I said. "There's nothing we can take away from him. And he likes to fight like this. I wish there were a hospital where we could put him, just for a week. It might give him a reason to try to control himself."

Tony stopped struggling and sat up in bed with a look of alarm in his eyes.

"Tony be good boy," he promised.

We stared at him in disbelief. My knees felt weak and I sat down on the bed with a laugh of relief. Tony wasn't possessed by some mysterious, uncontrollable, psychotic rage. Maybe we did have a way to teach him. Tony feared hospitals and for several years we used that fear.

He had his next tantrum while in the car and tried to kick out the windshield. I turned the car around and drove toward the hospital, telling Tony where we were going. Tony stopped kicking at the windshield and sat up in his seat. He pleaded with me to turn back, promising to be a good boy. We reached the hospital. We drove slowly by the emergency entrance, and Tony cried,

"Oh no, Tony's going to get a little new baby. No! No! Tony doesn't want a baby."

I couldn't resist laughing, which only increased Tony's alarm. I took him home. A few days later Tony again declared he didn't want a baby.

"Boys and men don't get babies," I said, "just ladies."

"And Rin-Tin-Tin?"

"Rin-Tin-Tin?"

"You know - Tippy Toes."

"Oh," I said with a laugh, "you mean Tiny Tim."

A newscaster had announced Tiny Tim, a male TV comedian who sang *Tip Toe Through the Tulips* in a falsetto voice, would become a father. No one had mentioned Tiny Tim's wife, Miss Vickie, would have the baby.

Tony behaved for a while, but about a year later he threw rocks and broke windows at school. I warned him doctors had an injection to cure boys of throwing rocks, and if he threw any more I'd have him inoculated. Terrified of shots, Tony behaved for a few weeks. Then one day his teacher phoned to say Tony had gone on a rampage, smashing all the dishes at school. I drove to school and got him. Tony didn't plead with me not to take him to the hospital. He seemed to realize the seriousness of his behavior and appeared resigned to endure the consequences. Once home I told him to pack his suitcase—in case the injection didn't work. Doctors might decide surgery was necessary, I added.

As we drove to the hospital, I kept waiting for Tony to beg me to turn back. He remained solemnly silent. We arrived at the emergency entrance. Unless he started begging to go home Tony was about to learn we had been bluffing for the past two years. Without some threat to control him, whatever could we do?

I parked the car, and we walked slowly into the emergency room. Tony was carrying his suitcase and courageously prepared to undergo his treatment. I glanced uneasily around the room and saw two nurses. They didn't seem busy.

"We want one of those inoculations to cure boys of throwing rocks," I finally requested, as I held up an index finger and winked frantically. At the same time I attempted what I hoped was a pleading expression on my face.

They stared at me—and at Tony, stoically carrying his suitcase. Finally a look of comprehension flooded across the face of the older nurse. She pricked Tony on the finger, and he screamed in agony. It was a powerful injection, curing him of throwing rocks for several years.

CHAPTER 17

What if patients wrote case histories about doctors?

In California, state agencies, called Regional Centers, are responsible for retarded people during their entire lives, providing appropriate services. Tony didn't need anything at the moment. We were thinking of his future when we applied for his acceptance by the Golden Gate Regional Center. We signed a release allowing them to send for his records. A doctor interviewed Ike and me, and decided a psychiatrist should evaluate Tony. The psychiatrist observed Tony briefly at school. When I met him in his office he said,

"Tony's teacher tells me you've written a book about your son. If I could read it, we might save time evaluating him."

I hesitated. Other doctors had read my manuscript, including most of those about whom I'd written. I'd even summoned the courage to return to the Child Guidance Clinic with it one day. Glancing uneasily around that familiar waiting room, the scene of unpleasant memories, Isaw the same assortment of mothers and children. A psychologist in a white coat was behind the reception desk arguing with someone on the phone.

That report was just our professional opinion," I overheard him declare defensively. "We regret you don't find our suggestions helpful."

I plopped my manuscript down upon the reception counter "I've written a book about you guys. If this wasn't what happened here, tell me what did," I said. "Call me when you finish reading it," I added and fled.

They kept my manuscript for a month, but someone finally phoned that they were finished with it. I returned apprehensively to the clinic, wondering if anyone might try to dispute my version of what had happened during those two and a half years. However, a psychologist handed my manuscript back with a stony, expressionless look on his face. "We have no comment," he said.

When Freud first proposed publishing case histories, the medical profession was horrified, accusing him of violating the confidential doctor patient relationship. Freud insisted revelation of skeletons in his patients' closets was quite acceptable so long as he didn't use real names. Psychiatrists had been publishing case histories ever since. None of the doctors' names in my book were real. Nevertheless, their reaction to my "case history" confounded me. Now this psychiatrist who was evaluating Tony for the Regional Center was *asking* to read my book. Since he apparently knew I'd written something, how could I refuse? A clinic at San Francisco State College had diagnosed Tony as retarded. He was attending classes for the retarded. I was secretary for Marin Aid to Retarded Children. Surely psychiatry no longer had any claim upon us. I took my book to the psychiatrist's office. After reading it, he phoned and said I needn't come for it. He left the manuscript in our mailbox early one morning.

I returned to talk to the doctor at the Regional Center. She said Tony could not obtain services from the agency. "Your son is not retarded. He's schizophrenic," she said.

"Schizophrenic!" I repeated. "How did you make that diagnosis?"

"Retarded children don't have the superior nervous system your son has." The first day we came to the Regional Center, the doctor had asked Tony to draw a boy. Tony, always impatient to be done with doctors, quickly drew a boy with a penis, five fingers on each hand and five toes on each foot, without lifting the pencil from the paper. The doctor had commented such a feat was difficult for normal children and indicated an undamaged nervous system. (I doubt Tony's nervous system is still superior. He has been taught to print his name, and does so crudely and laboriously.)

"May I talk to the psychiatrist who made the diagnosis?" I asked.

"That won't be necessary," the doctor replied uneasily. "I diagnosed him myself. We merely asked the psychiatrist to confirm my opinion." She made it plain she didn't wish to discuss Tony's schizophrenia.

I went home and phoned the psychiatrist. "I understand you believe my son is schizophrenic," I said. "May I make an appointment to discuss his diagnosis?"

"No," he answered, "That would not accomplish anything."

The psychiatrist had evaluated Tony for a state agency. He was paid by tax money. Nevertheless I did not argue. I'd learned how helpless I was against the medical profession. Doctors and government agencies apparently felt entitled to use such diagnoses however they chose, with no obligation to explain anything. I remembered the child psychiatrist I'd consulted some years before, the doctor who advised me to go tell Dr. Dingle "exactly what I thought of him", the charming psychiatrist who only charged me half-price for that advice. He had seemed like an intelligent, forthright man. I phoned him for another appointment.

As I again seated myself in the psychiatrist's big comfortable chair and glanced through the plate glass window at the small-boat harbor, I explained I'd consulted him several years before. This time I didn't want to discuss my child, I said, I wished to inquire about the general subjects of autism and childhood schizophrenia.

"Autism is one of my specialties," he said.

Then I guess you've read Dr. Bernard Rimland's book, *Early Infantile Autism?*"

"Well, no," he answered.

I was taken aback. Dr. Rimland had an autistic son, and was one the founders of the National Society for Autistic Children. His book had questioned whether maternal rejection could cause autism, but it was the only scholarly, factual book I'd found in this country on the subject. It had won a scientific award. I couldn't imagine why anyone concerned with autism hadn't read it. I had sent to England for books and asked if the psychiatrist had read those.

He had not.

Surely a psychiatrist claiming a specialty in autism must have read something on the subject. I asked if he'd read publications I had been unable to locate. He mentioned a scientific paper written a decade before and offered to obtain a copy for me.

"Do you still believe children become abnormal because of something in their environment?" I asked.

He smiled and shook his head.

"No, many of my views on child psychiatry have changed in the past few years."

Someone once said: "Obsolete ideas don't fade away; their proponents just die off." In the interest of stability, nature seemed to have made flexibility a trait of the young. A psychiatrist who could discard beliefs to which he had devoted much of his life might be the reasonable, open-minded doctor for whom I'd been searching. *If only I could persuade him to talk to me!* I told him I'd written a book about Tony, adding I'd described my consultation with him some years earlier.

"Have you!"

"Would you like to read it?"

"I certainly would," he answered. "I'll call you when I finish," he promised, as he took the manuscript and began leafing through it with interest. My naturally optimistic nature surged. Rational discussion seemed so simple and easy. To my knowledge, this psychiatrist was not part of any government clinic or public agency. (I was mistaken about him not being a part of a public agency. He was on the board of directors of the nursery school where I was told Tony could attend, only if he were under the care of a psychiatrist. The psychiatrist who told the Regional Center Tony was schizophrenic, and then refused to discuss his diagnosis, was on the same board of directors. However I didn't learn any of this until many years later.)

A month passed before the psychiatrist phoned me to return for my manuscript. "Just knock on my inner office door if I'm busy," he said. Arriving at the appointed hour, excited with anticipation, I knocked. A muffled "just a moment" sounded from within. There was a chair by the door, and I sat down. Presently the door opened a few inches, and I watched as the psychiatrist's head and one arm with my manuscript appeared.

"Well, er—ah, thank you," he stammered, handing me the envelope. His head and arm disappeared and the door snapped closed.

Unable to move, I stared at the door. Apparently the psychiatrist had changed his mind about the scientific paper he had promised. *Why?* There was nothing unflattering about him in my book! The effort to face myself at the typewriter had sometimes been painful. Anyone who writes must be willing to appear naked. Vanities and unintentional dishonesties are often revealed for the first time when a writer sees them on paper. One difficult task had been to separate what I actually said to doctors from what I later wished I had said. Nevertheless I was confident I had remembered my conversation with this psychiatrist accurately enough. I sat staring at the closed door, again immobilized by frustration as I slammed against the mysterious, invisible wall that prevented doctors from talking to me. After so many disappointments, I must not allow another one to evoke such painful feelings, I told myself. Finally, I got up from the chair and went home to cope with my anger at yet another doctor. The bill the psychiatrist sent me that time was full price.

Since doctors refused to talk to me, I read everything I could find about atypical children. Convinced government research was responsible for doctors' strange behavior, I wondered if autism might be discussed more rationally in other countries. I sent for scientific papers in German and asked a German friend to make sure I translated them correctly. Although I found plenty of esoteric discussion about damaged psyches, published facts about autism or childhood schizophrenia in any language were meager and unenlightening. Several popular books on autism seemed preposterous. One widely read account was made into a movie. The author claimed to have cured his autistic son by some vague form of "love" and constant attention. His method of treatment proposed that a therapist non-judgmentally enter the child's private world of autism. Then the autistic child should be invited, politely, to come out and join the real world.

How could the medical profession take such nonsense seriously?

Bruno Bettelheim, a columnist for *Ladies Home Journal,* was notorious among parents of autistic children for claiming maternal rejection caused autism. He was one of the first to expound the theory that a "real person" had been hiding in the body of each autistic child, afraid to come out. According to Bettelheim, in the first weeks of life, during bonding, a baby might decide mother was rejecting it. "Ah-ha," the tiny infant might cleverly reason, "Mother is out to exterminate me! But if I don't exist mother will be unable to destroy me." Bettelheim speculated this was the moment when a baby decides to become autistic.

Faced with such preposterous theories, my faith in the pronouncements of "scientific authorities" continued to deteriorate. Many of the people who were taking such theories seriously were not ignorant. The medical profession was, supposedly, the most critical, scientifically educated segment of our society, and most of us assumed they were not gullible.

I often tried to expunge from my mind the belief that we were vic- tims of some secret research program. Believing only what one wishes must be a comforting ability. Nevertheless, I would wake up one morn- ing and find the belief had taken over my head like some big unwelcome monster. I remembered that psychoanalysis was launched by a secret, international conspiracy.

After the first decade of this century, Freud and his little group of fel- low psychoanalysts in Vienna were still regarded with scorn and deri- sion by most of the world. Jung and Adler had been excommunicated from "The Movement" for suggesting neurosis and mental illness might be caused by something other than infantile sex and Oedipus com- plexes. Such treachery caused well-documented emotional trauma among faithful Freudian analysts. Entire books have been written describing the emotional trauma Freud suffered at Jung's defection. In 1912 Freud's disciples organized an international committee to be on guard against further heresies. Freud insisted this committee be kept secret; knowledge of its existence might further damage their already unsavory public image. For the next ten years they were vigilant in stamping out deviant ideas about psychoanalysis. Finally Freudian analysis was imposed upon Western society (mostly in the US) as sci- ence, and the committee could be publicly acknowledged.

I did finally emerge from an encounter with psychiatry feeling tri- umphant rather than defeated. It occurred some years later and in, of all places, Freud's hometown, Vienna.

After my husband died, and when Tony began attending a camp for retarded children every summer, I discovered a fascinating way to travel. I would go to a foreign country and enroll in a language school. I had spent a wonderful summer with five other women, living in a dormitory at the *Cite Universitaire* in Paris, and studying French at the *Sorbonne*. A couple of summers later I went alone to Vienna and studied German at the *Goethe Institute*. My classmates were European businessmen, diplomats, aspiring young opera singers, bright young priests, college professors, and students from all over the world. The language classes were stimulating, but I was even more fascinated by my fellow students. Many of their lives were quite different from mine, and I loved talking to people with diverse beliefs and attitudes. The *Goethe Institute* didn't offer much organized social life, so I appointed myself an unofficial social director that summer and arranged trips on the Danube and to the Vienna Woods. We spent evenings in the wine gardens of Grinzing. The young people appreciated the outings I organized, and we became good friends.

One evening we missed the last streetcar from Grinzing and had to walk back to Vienna. The party included a young Swedish couple with a baby in a stroller. It as a lovely summer night, and the conversation was interesting. We arrived back in Vienna in pre-dawn hours, the baby sleeping soundly. Vienna was a quiet, old-fashioned city. Teenage boys on streetcars even got up and gave their seat to a lady. Strangers spoke to each other on the street. "*Gruss Gott,*" was the greeting I returned as I approached my hotel along the dark, almost deserted sidewalk. Being out alone in a large city at such a late hour, without fear, reminded me of San Francisco when I was young. This enchanting city was where psychiatry began. This was where Freud and his disciples dreamed up all those weird theories that had plagued me for two decades.

I was in an advanced language class. Viennese professionals lectured on various topics, which we discussed in German. Some of the subjects were controversial and the discussions lively. One such lecturer had advanced degrees in philosophy and psychology, and touched upon the subject of child psychiatry and maternal rejection.

"How can you define maternal rejection?" I challenged him, my German word order becoming somewhat tangled in my indignation. "How can any psychologist presume to judge whether a mother loves her child!"

The polite, mild-spoken Austrian lecturer stared at me in consternation. I apologized for my outburst, and he asked if he might continue. Going on to name illnesses caused by maternal rejection, he placed autism at the top of the list. I was silent, but the expression on my face must have been explosive.

I visited Hungary alone the weekend after that incident. As I explored the twin cities of Buda and Pest, connected by bridges across the Danube, my mind kept returning to the lecturer in Vienna. In the United States hardly anyone except Bruno Bettelheim still believed maternal rejection caused autism. But in Vienna, the very cradle of psychiatry, such an outdated view persisted.

It was a cold, drizzly weekend. Buying some paper, I spent Sunday afternoon in a deserted, outdoor cafe by the silent, gray Danube. Oblivious to the weather, I sat writing my own lecture on autism, in German. Many facts were in my head. (I brazenly made up one.) I told how autism was first defined by Dr. Leo Kanner in 1945. After the election of John Kennedy, who had a retarded sister, massive research efforts were undertaken on atypical children. Summarizing the literature, I described attempts to treat autism with psychiatry, and told of the parents' rebellion against this treatment. "Traditional theories have been disproved by soon-to-be-released research results," I stated. (This was the part I made up.)

Returning to Vienna by train, I shared a compartment with some young Austrians. They allowed me to practice my lecture, showing a lively interest in the subject and correcting my German. Monday morning the Austrian lecturer brought a colleague with him to class, another psychologist.

Good, I thought. If he was seeking moral support in case I disrupted the class again, I would enlighten them both! I asked if I might give a short talk, for dissertations by students were part of the instruction. I had managed to overcome much of my shyness, and could talk to strangers informally. However, my knees would have ordinarily been shaking, and my voice quivering with fear at the prospect of standing up and speaking before an audience, even an audience of friends. Nevertheless, on this particular day, I forgot all stage fright. My report was magnificent, and my German flawless. Everyone in the room appeared convinced, including the two psychologists, and eagerly questioned me on the subject I had so confidently presented.

I sure fixed you, Freud, you old rascal, I thought gleefully, and in your own home town! For that one brief moment I didn't feel so isolated with my bothersome, research-conspiracy theory.

CHAPTER 18

A Mexican cure for profanity

I wish I could report we lived happily ever after, all troubles behind us. If such bliss were ever achieved, I suspect many people would be tempted to invent a few problems out of boredom, (the real reason Adam and Eve decided to escape from that garden) but I never found myself faced with the predicament.

Ike was nine years older than I, and for fifty-six years he led a reasonably happy life. His last five years were not happy. His health deteriorated. Ike blamed his drinking, about which he had always felt guilty. He developed emphysema, but was unable to stop smoking. Although Ike always did his best, I think Tony's retardation also became too much for him. We each have limits. Ike had been a wonderful husband and father. Now, feeling defeated, he seemed to lose interest in everything and withdrew from life. He died after surgery on an ulcer, which had remained undiagnosed in spite of frequent medical examinations. I had already spent five years grieving for him, unable to help as I watched him lose interest in life. One of my deepest sorrows is how unhappy Ike's last few years were.

About a year after Ike's death, I got around to thinking about what Tony and I might do with our lives. It had become obvious Tony would never achieve much independence, even with special education. I decided to live in Mexico, where Tony and I could live together, and inexpensive help might give me some freedom. I sold my house, and Sherry, Tony and I drove leisurely down to Guadalajara. Tony enjoyed Mexico, and the Mexicans often seemed to enjoy him.

"He doesn't have any worries, does he?" exclaimed one Mexican with a laugh of admiration.

At fifteen, the number of things Tony feared was not yet great, and he still had an appetite for new experiences. Near a motel in Mazatlan, where we stopped for a few days, workmen were digging a well. They would lower a bucket into the hole and fill it with dirt. Then they would walk out into a field with the end of the rope, pulling up the bucket. One day we heard cheering at the well. Tony was pulling up the bucket as the Mexican workmen applauded. When we left they all came and waved goodbye to him.

At that time I'd been unable to restrain Tony from swearing. When he realized everyone was speaking another language, he begged us to tell him some dirty words in Spanish. Finally, with exaggerated reluctance we agreed, warning him to never repeat them.

Tony promised, with his mischievous little grin and familiar impish sparkle in his eye.

"*Buenos Dios* is the most terrible thing anyone can say in Spanish," we confided.

Tony mischievously ran up and exclaimed "*Buenos Dios!*" to everyone. Most Mexicans reacted with surprise, and while it wasn't the outrage Tony's profanity usually evoked, it was apparently enough of a reaction to satisfy Tony. We pretended anger, scolding him and punishing him by denying him dessert when he said the forbidden words. Tony became fascinated with his new profanity and forgot all English swear words.

I rented an apartment in Guadalajara, and Sherry returned to college in the States. I made friends with the Americans living there and hired a Mexican woman to watch Tony. One afternoon I suggested Maria take him shopping while I played bridge. Maria thought I said Tony would take her shopping. Happy for someone to obediently follow him, Tony led her all over Guadalajara. I wondered who was watching whom. Nevertheless Tony was becoming more responsible, and I didn't worry.

Tony loved Guadalajara, enjoying the music, the parks, the food, and shopping in the big colorful, crowded markets. Mexicans drive like rodeo cowboys, and the bus ride to town was always wild and exciting. We joined a sports club and went swimming every morning. I took a painting class, held in a park where a karate class was also taking place. Tony laughed with delight as the karate students yelled and leaped. A willow tree in front of our apartment provided plenty of the limber sticks Tony liked to shake. A music group practiced in a nearby house. Tony, an enthralled listener, spent balmy evenings on the sidewalk, contentedly shaking his stick. No one tried to make Tony talk in Guadalajara, and I'd never seen him happier.

Tony's emotional episodes usually came unexpectedly. One evening he refused to go to bed, staying up all night and laughing in a way that did not suggest humor. He lost his temper often, and sometimes became defiant. One morning we were shopping in a big produce market. Persistent little Mexican boys aggressively competed to carry shopping baskets, jumping on cars several blocks from the market and fighting to be hired. I always gave one a peso to avoid harassment from the others. My Mexican boy, in addition to carrying my basket, was busy fending off attacks from his tough little competitors. As I was leaving the market on this particular morning, having paid off my little helper, I looked around for Tony and saw him surrounded by policemen. They seemed to be fighting with him, bending his arm behind his back. I dropped my produce and ran back. I tried to persuade them to allow Tony to get into my car, and then tell me what he'd done. In my fright I forgot how to speak Spanish. I couldn't remember the words to explain Tony was retarded. One of the policemen kept insisting Tony was "a very dangerous fellow".

They finally allowed him to get in the car and stood guard over him, their hands hovering over their pistols. One of them took me to the police station, where someone spoke English. The police captain was apologetic when he learned Tony was retarded, but I forgot to ask what he'd done. Perhaps something happened between him and one of the little Mexican boys. Tony was twice their size. He was bigger than the policemen.

Shaken, I rushed back to the market. *Oh why did such a thing have to happen to Tony!* He might need help someday, and I didn't want him to fear the police. But as was often the case, Tony's reaction was not what I expected. He thought the police were playing with him.

"Tell about the time Tony wrestled eight Mexican policemen," he would gleefully urge me to repeat the story for several years afterwards. He tried to entice men in uniform into another wrestling match.

Nevertheless the episode terrified me. I decided a foreign country was a dangerous place for a big, strange acting boy who didn't look retarded. Frantic to return to the States, I packed the car. A fan belt broke. A mechanic patched it, but said I should order a new one before starting on the long journey to California. He phoned Loredo, Texas, and ordered it put on a bus, saying it would arrive *manana*. According to a Spanish dictionary *manana* means tomorrow, but in Mexico it obviously means "some time in the future". For two weeks I returned to the garage every morning with all my possessions in the car, and was told "*manana*". Tony became more upset. I felt alone and terrified, as though I were living on top of a bomb. A long-distance phone call to California would have been difficult and complicated, and Guy and Sherry were unaware of our trouble. However Sherry later said she had a dream in which she saw me sitting onthe side of the bed crying. That was how I spent many of my nights during those two weeks.

The part for the car finally came and we drove back to California. Tony returned to the same class for retarded children he'd been attending six months earlier. Within a few weeks he recovered from his emotional upset.

That broken fan belt, which allowed Tony to recover from him emotional upset naturally, protected him from anti-psychotic drugs for three more years.

During that time I managed to create a good life for Tony and me. He attended classes for trainable 'retarded' children. The little yellow bus picked him up every morning. On weekends he participated in Easter Seals recreation programs for the handicapped. He became so responsible I sometimes left him alone in the evening. I took courses at a community college. On days when Tony wasn't in school, he played on campus while waiting for me. For ten weeks every summer he attended a camp for retarded children, which gave me opportunity to travel. Guy and Sherry no longer lived at home, but we saw them often.

Just as I was again deciding we'd overcome all our problems, my world suddenly became unraveled once more. One day at school Tony was working in the garden. He lifted his rake and hit the boy next to him on the head, wounding him so seriously as to require stitches. Tony had never been aggressive. He had thrown rocks at windows and broken things, but he had never struck anyone. When asked why he'd done such a thing, Tony replied,

"Because I was mad."

"Why were you mad?" we persisted.

Tony merely shook his head. It was a reason that, to him, needed no explanation. Tony was nineteen years old. The school system was no longer required to provide an education program, and he had to stay home. He seemed to be going through a particularly bad time, losing control every few days. I was afraid to take him anywhere and I was afraid to leave him alone. We both stayed in the apartment. Tony had nothing to do but lie in bed and eat. He gained twenty pounds.

For years the threat of my baby in an institution had horrified me. I'd planned to decide where he would live as an adult before he became too old to adjust easily. Tony was still childlike however, and I thought of him becoming a man sometime in the future. Now I had to find a place for him, and no one had any suggestions except the state hospital. I visited the hospital and found it depressing. The buildings and grounds were nice enough, and the people working there seemed kind. Nevertheless it's painful for normal people to look at large groups of severely handicapped individuals, regardless of the setting. Perhaps such experiences fill us with guilt about our own seemingly more satisfactory lives. I had managed to cope with Tony's problems for nineteen years. His commitment to the state hospital seemed an admission of tragic failure.

Both Guy and Sherry were also having problems. Guy, for some years near the head of his class at the university, was in graduate school. Suddenly surrounded by the brightest young physicists in the country, he was feeling inadequate. Furthermore he was a teaching assistant, trying to teach the only class in which he'd done poorly as an undergraduate. Some of his students knew as much about his subject matter as he did. Sherry was having difficulty in nursing training. She did well academically, but her superiors kept telling her she wasn't assertive enough to deal with doctors and become a nurse. I understood, for I had once feared doctors and been unassertive myself. It was the first year of the great drought in California, but it was a damp spring around our house. I shed tears about Tony; Sherry wept because she feared she wouldn't become a nurse; Guy, with problems of his own, tried to console us.

In California parents can't apply for their child's admission to a state hospital; application must be made by a social worker. I was unable to move my social workers to action. They called meetings to discuss Tony, always coming to the conclusion the state hospital was the best place for him. No one got around to filling out the papers. Instead, they called more meetings. Perhaps they were intentionally deliberate to prevent parents from making impulsive decisions, but I felt frustrated and was again reminded that psychologists and social workers felt their role was to manipulate people.

After several months Tony was finally admitted to a program for autistic boys, a special, experimental program at the hospital. He lived in a cottage with about thirty young men. I brought him home on weekends and soon realized Tony enjoyed living there. Like any nineteen-year-old, he considered a cottage full of young men more fun than living in an apartment with Mom! I visited Tony, and we went to the hospital snack bar. A patient at a nearby table was talking to himself, gesturing and laughing out loud. Tony laughed too. I suppose he found such bizarre behavior more interesting than the sedate world of normal people.

One weekend I brought Tony home, and he asked if Guy and Sherry were coming to dinner. I said no. He asked if we were going to visit Grandmother. Again I said no, not this weekend.

"Then why did you bring me home?" he asked.

He wanted to return to the hospital for a dance that evening, so I took him back. He ran into the cottage, laughing and yelling, "I'm here! I'm here!"

Tony lived at the hospital for two years. The social workers and teachers seemed dedicated. Most professionals dealing with the retarded are people with tolerance and compassion. For a while Tony attended a special education class at the local high school near the hospital. One day he became bored and pulled all the fire alarms, bringing fire engines screeching to the school. That ended his main streaming. He didn't feel much desire to do things normal people do, and was just as happy attending the class held at the hospital.

Professionals concerned with the handicapped wanted to close state hospitals, feeling retarded people should live in the community. A California law stated any patient asking to leave in front of witnesses must be released or granted a court hearing. Some of the young men were smart enough to learn they could create excitement by demanding to leave. In Tony's case, I suspect a social worker who believed in community placements put him up to it. Since Tony seemed happy there, I preferred the safety of an institution. Nevertheless, Tony was placed in a group home in San Francisco with five retarded young men. Medication was supposed to control his disruptive behavior. He attended a day program for the handicapped. I soon realized Tony would be happy wherever he lived. Maybe he inherited my cheerful nature.

Many mothers have trouble redefining themselves after their youngest child leaves home, and being the mother of a handicapped child is an intense experience. Sherry became a nurse, and Guy got his Ph.D. They were all living their own lives. None of them, including Tony, had much need for me any more. Some independent, grown children, and my children were independent, might resent their parents not having a life of their own. I was determined not to try to live the rest of my life through my children. Having survived my traumatic encounter with the medical profession, I was confident I could do anything. It seemed a little late to start a career. Besides, with my Army pension I had enough money to live as I always had.

Rather than sit around waiting for old age, I finally decided to try to live my favorite fantasy.

CHAPTER 19

Is Western culture "normal"?

During that bleak night in 1961, when Ike was in Greenland, and I struggled alone to accept Tony's retardation, I remember believing happiness was gone forever, and that my life had become a tragedy. The truth is, raising a handicapped child could never diminish anyone's life. Coping was a challenge while Tony was growing up, but those were not unhappy years. Contrary to twentieth-century dogma, surviving traumatic events does not "damage" our psyches; it can even stimulate our growth, adding value to our lives. As a result of resisting the psychologists, I had lost much of my shyness. I was in my late fifties as I set out on my new venture, a woman no longer easily intimidated by everyone except small children and other housewives.

My favorite fantasy had always been to travel around the world in a sailboat. Personal accounts by such sailors were my favorite reading. I also lived my own adventures. I cut a picture of my boat from a sailing magazine. Plotting my daily mileage on a map, in knots, I planned lists of provisions and found books in the library describing the exotic places I visited.

We once took the children and some of their friends for a two-week houseboat vacation on Lake Shasta. The houseboat rental company sent us a big map of the lake. I traced it, renaming campsites Patagonia, Ceylon and Zanzibar. Warnings of fantastic dangers, such as pirates, headhunters, wars and mythical beasts covered my map. I tacked it up on the bulkhead of the houseboat, and we all amused ourselves by pretending we were visiting such exotic places, instead of "Eel River Camp" or "Pine Flat". The houseboat broke down in "Bora Bora". The children paddled their inner tubes to "Australia" for help, evading "Fiji cannibals" along the way. When the vacation was over I suggested leaving our map on the boat for someone else to enjoy. The children were at an age where they couldn't tolerate being thought different. Embarrassed for the world to learn about Mother's extravagant imagination, they indignantly took down the map.

Guy and Sherry were adults now, and expressed interested approval when I announced I was leaving to travel around the world. (By more conventional means than a sailboat, I hasten to add.) Tony's destructiveness had convinced me possessions were unimportant, and I didn't have much of value. Giving up my apartment, I stored a couple of boxes of personal belongings in a friend's basement. I'd already learned traveling and living in foreign countries doesn't have to be more expensive than living in California. My Army pension could go directly to my checking account, and an American Express card allowed me to obtain cash in most countries of the world.

I had already discovered lone travelers do face one danger: a debilitating feeing of isolation. Always self-sufficient, my need for a certain amount of social interaction had surprised me. A few years earlier, during my first trip to Europe (while Tony was at summer camp) I'd found I wasn't having as much fun as I had expected. Being continually surrounded by people, but having no personal relationship with anyone, had caused a strange, heavy feeling. During my encounters with doctors, I had felt grief, fear, indignation and anger. I coped with such feelings by expressing them to family and friends, and at the typewriter. Traveling alone in Europe was my first experience with depression.

I took a day cruise in the Balearic Islands. The other tourists on the boat were French, Spanish and Italian. I was aware of people glancing uncertainly at me, the only person not speaking to anyone. Probably no one knew which language to use. Ordinarily I'd have been delighted to attempt all three, but in my despondent perversity I refused to utter a word. I had become so isolated I spurned friendly overtures. Aborting my vacation, I returned home.

Back among family and friends I tried to understand what had happened to me, and how to prevent it from happening again. I determinedly tried another trip. I'd probably never be capable of scintillating small talk at a cocktail party, but I did force myself to learn to approach strangers and to interact with them on a personal level.

Friends had expressed awe at the courage required for a woman to travel alone. I couldn't deny a feeling of apprehension as I boarded the plane for Hong Kong, but this was to be the great adventure of my life, and excitement outweighed fear. One of the fears people had mentioned was arriving in a strange country without a hotel reservation. In Hong Kong, my first stop, I spent one night in an expensive, first class hotel. Such hotels always have available rooms, I'd discovered, but price is not the only reason to avoid them. Guests in first class hotels don't talk to strangers. Conversations with people traveling on the cheap come easier. Most such travelers are young, bright and curious. Those who are older seem to have retained that curiosity. One wouldn't think of getting into a philosophical discussion with someone in the supermarket line at home, but such discussions feel unremarkable with some traveler you'll probably never see again.

The day after my arrival in Hong Kong, I rented a room at the Kowloon YMCA, across the street from the Star Ferry. There I found adventurous, approachable travelers from all over the world. Evenings we sat in the tea garden on the roof and watched the lights of Hong

Kong across Victoria Harbor. Sailboats, fishing boats, freighters, barges, junks, *san pans*, ferries and hydrofoils scurried about, miraculously avoiding collisions.

A tour seemed a prudent way for a lone woman to experience local nightlife, and *Hong-Kong-by-Night* included dinner at an Aberdeen floating restaurant and a nightclub performance of Chinese opera. My companions were French and Portuguese tourists, and I practiced talking French with them. The Chinese tour guide spoke only English, with a very proper British accent. During the evening he explained most residents of Hong Kong were proud to be British colonials, with no desire for independence. New construction was everywhere, and our guide expressed a veritable reverence for private enterprise. In 1997 China was scheduled to regain the colony when a ninety-nine-year lease expired. The guide assured us private enterprise had spent millions in Hong Kong, and China wouldn't dare retake it. He was also certain China would not develop tourist facilities for many years. "How could they accomplish such a thing without private enterprise?"

Pamphlets describing bus and ferry routes made it easy for tourists to get around in Hong Kong, and one day I boarded a municipal bus for the northern mainland area. We passed through towns, their narrow streets lined with tall apartment buildings. Laundry hung on long poles stuck out from each window, seeming to almost meet overhead and obscure the sky. Hundreds of identically dressed children were on their way to school. Their uniform included a gleaming white shirt, a necktie and a jacket with a school emblem on the pocket. They looked very British.

I enjoyed temples and other sights, but was also eager for something more than the usual tourist experience. At lunchtime I got off the bus to look for a real Chinese restaurant, one where only Chinese ate. The one I chose was enormous, two stories high and a quarter of a block square, and filled with noisy patrons. A waiter, threading a way through the tightly packed chairs and big round tables, found a place for me at a table with seven other people. The appearance of a Western woman caused them to stop talking for about sixty seconds. Then they resumed their noisy babble. The waiter didn't speak English, so I pointed to something on the menu. My food, when it arrived, looked strange and tasted awful. The din of Chinese voices rang in my ears. Across the table a woman was holding a baby with *Dienstag*, German for Tuesday, embroidered on it's bib. The baby was chewing on a big gray chicken claw. As the only Westerner in the room, I must have looked conspicuous, but the Chinese were too polite to stare. They continued laughing, talking and eating. I began to experience an unpleasant sensation of being invisible in that huge room full of noisy Chinese. I waved for the waiter and gave him some money. Dumping the change in my purse, I left.

I boarded a bus to return to Kowloon. A good-looking, blond young man sat down next to me. He wore a coat and tie, and his hair was short and neatly combed. It had been years since I'd noticed an American kid looking so well groomed. He must surely be a British resident, I decided.

Then a warning bell went off in my head. I was feeling hesitant about initiating conversation with the boy. My experience in the restaurant had caused feelings of isolation, feelings I knew could grow, and I'd better start talking to someone soon, or my adventure might fail before I got much further

"Are you visiting Hong Kong or are you a resident?" I finally made myself ask.

"A little of both," he answered with an American, Western accent, and explained he was a Mormon missionary from Utah.

"Have you made many converts in Hong Kong?"

"None," he replied with a good-natured grin. "Some of these people are Buddhists and some practice a form of ancestor worship. Actually, most people in Hong Kong seem to worship money," he added wryly.

"I've noticed their admiration for private enterprise," I agreed with amusement.

Like most of the young people I met, he appeared eager to talk, and explained most Mormon boys spend a year on a mission. After learning the language, he had visited Chinese families to talk about his religion. Most had listened with polite interest. Now it was almost time for the young missionary to return to the States.

"And then what are your plans?" I asked.

"I love living in Hong Kong," he said, "and would like to come back. Chinese is a difficult language but I speak it fluently now. Maybe I'll go back to college and get a degree in business administration. I might get a job with some American company doing business here."

He was a delightful, intelligent young man, and I agreed he probably could. I doubt he realized one might claim he was converting to "private enterprise", the religion of the natives he'd been sent to Hong Kong to save.

While Hong Kong might hold some dangers for missionaries, there didn't seem to be anything that might threaten a woman of my age. On the other hand, Thailand, the next country in which I spent a few weeks, turned out to pose a possible danger for Italians. I witnessed a near clash between cultures, and who is to say which culture is more "normal". I emerged from the plane into the heat and humidity of Bangkok. The French tourists in Hong Kong had recommended an inexpensive hotel across the street from the huge, endlessly fascinating outdoor market. There one could buy live frogs and geese, plastic combs, pig's heads, beautiful straw hats, rayon underpants, bronze Buddhas, tiny birds plucked of feathers and ready to cook, orchids, edible insects and other strange objects. There were no other Americans at the hotel, and I usually found myself with Europeans on local tours. Once, on a crowded bus, I got into a conversation with a New Zealander, a member of his House of Parliament. Among other things, he explained that lawyers and lawsuits had been almost eliminated in his country by a prohibition against collecting money for 'pain and suffering'.

"I wonder where we ever got the idea that 'pain and suffering' was something for which people were entitled to financial compensation? People once accepted 'pain and suffering' as a normal part of life," I commented. "I know one thing, though," I told the New Zealander. "No American politician would sit down on a bus and talk to some ordinary tourist sitting next to him as you are doing. Members of our congress have voted themselves huge salaries, and would probably expect to be driven around in limousines."

"In New Zealand a politician displaying more wealth than his constituents wouldn't be re-elected," he said.

I felt I had made extraordinary progress in initiating conversations with strangers. Here I was discussing policy with members of foreign governments!

The most pleasant way to get around Bangkok was by ferry and water taxi. From the street the Thai capital was hot, drab, congested and ugly, but from the water it was lovely. Temples, hidden behind high walls, exposed their golden splendor to the *klongs* and other waterways. Intricately carved teak houses could be glimpsed among the vegetation along the banks. Some had colorful, steep, tile roofs and some were thatched. Even shacks with rusty, tin roofs looked picturesque amidst the trees and tropical plants. The people along the rivers seemed to live half in the water, like exotic amphibians. They swam in their sarongs and washed their hair, clothes and food in the river. Water buffalo stood motionless in the cool water as children splashed around them. Ferries ran like streetcars, and women in canoes sold produce, flowers and hot cooked food.

The attractive Thai people displayed a serene manner, considering anger a sin. (Western psychologists would surely regard them as repressed.) They sat patiently in the traffic jams of Bangkok, neither swearing nor honking horns, as people do in most big cities of the world. I'd read that Thai people also had an aversion, understandable in that climate, to being touched. Not fond of being touched, myself, I was glad to hear that somewhere the feeling was regarded as "normal". (Aversion to being touched had been mentioned as one of the pathologies of autism.)

On a sightseeing trip down the river, the guide told us that a century ago the penalty for touching the king or a member of the royal family had been death. He related a pathetic little story about three royal children who drowned because of this Thai tabu. The children were out in a boat alone, and it tipped over. People stood on shore and watched them drown, rather than touch them.

After a couple of weeks I booked a Golden Triangle tour to northern Thailand. The corner where Thailand, Burma and Laos meet receives its name from the opium poppies grown there. I became friendly with a likeable young Italian on the same tour. His culture included lots of touching. He was a gentleman and never did anything more than pat the shoulder of our pretty little Thai tour guide, or lay his hand on her arm, as he did to everyone. Nevertheless I watched her cringe at his friendly gestures.

We rode elephants as they worked a teak forest. We visited an opium-smoking tribe, a dirty, dull eyed, pathetic looking group who augmented their poppy growing industry by selling beads and trinkets to tourists. European explorers, during the last century, sold beads and trinkets to natives all over the world. Who would have guessed natives would someday sell so many beads and trinkets back to European tourists.

One afternoon we were on a mountain road visiting a Buddhist temple. Several truckloads of soldiers with rifles came and announced the King would pass by shortly. They ordered us to stand by the side of the road, with our hats off, and await the royal car. The Italian was talking to our tour guide. I noticed the soldiers' sullen glances as he repeatedly touched her. Then he did something that outraged them. He reached over and patted her on the head. He would have probably attracted less attention if he had patted her where Italians are reputed to pat girls. To a Thai, the head is the temple of the soul, and to touch it is an insult. The Thai soldiers muttered angrily among themselves and glared at the Italian. They advanced menacingly toward us with their rifles in their hands. Controlling their anger, they only ordered us to move back further. The Italian remained oblivious to the idea anyone had an urge to shoot him.

That evening I went to dinner with the Italian. He did wish he could find some spaghetti, instead of all this rice, but we were unsuccessful. As we were eating our rice he asked,

"Aren't your children concerned about you traveling alone to uncivilized corners of the world? I'd sure worry if my mother decided to go off and ride elephants in a Thai jungle."

"My children don't worry," I said with a laugh. "They are convinced their mother is invincible."

Having summoned the courage to face hostile psychologists, I wasn't finding much to fear in a Thai jungle. My children sensed my confidence.

From Thailand I flew to Nepal, a tiny kingdom in the Himalayas. It was the dry season and everything was brown and dusty. I was joining an overland bus tour in Katmandu, and had a reservation at the hotel from which the tour was to start. I shared a taxi from the airport with some young Australians. It was a rusty old vehicle of Indian make, the stuffing bulging out of the seats. The starter didn't work, and two drivers were required, one to steer and another to push. We would drive a few blocks, then cut the motor and coast, keeping both drivers busy. The Nepalese were under the impression this method of driving conserved petrol. At the hotel I learned my room wouldn't be available until the next day. For that first night, I was consigned to the dormitory, a sort of penthouse on the roof. Cots were lined up next to each other, and sleeping thus in a room full of strangers was a new experience. We were warned to keep the windows closed to prevent monkeys from stealing our belongings. Finally I'd arrived in a country so exotic monkeys ran wild.

The next morning a dozen brown monkeys scampered away as we came out onto the roof. More played on the brown dusty roofs surrounding us. While planning my trip during the past year, I had tried to learn something about the places I would visit. As I looked out over the quiet little mountain capital, Nepal's comic-opera history seemed more believable than it had when I'd researched it at home. For centuries the kings of Nepal married two queens in one ceremony. This custom caused endless palace intrigue, as both queens and their assorted offspring vied for power. A particularly bloody episode occurred at the middle of the nineteenth century, when half the nobility of Nepal was massacred. A young army officer seized power and declared himself Prime Minister. He and his descendants ruled Nepal for the next century, keeping the royal family captive in the palace. All Westerners were excluded from the little country, and radios and newspapers were prohibited. In the 1950's the young captive king escaped to India. Organizing a successful revolt, he returned to rule his country, keeping the Prime Minister prisoner in his home. The new king accepted Western financial aid and built the first road into the capital. Until then everyone had arrived in Katmandu on foot. A funky rope-pulley arrangement had hauled freight over the mountains into the little city.

Because of the rugged terrain and Nepal's long isolation from Western civilization, the tribes of the little kingdom remained separate, each with its own language and customs. I'd read that among some mountain people, a woman could have two husbands if they were brothers. Among some jungle tribes near the Indian border, a man might marry a woman only from a tribe to the east of his village. The fate of the men in the eastern-most village was not mentioned.

Amid chickens, ducks, goats and cows on the rocky, unpaved streets of Katmandu, walked Mongolian looking mountain people in colorful costumes and furs, holy men wearing nothing but a dingy cloth around their loins, women in bright silk saris, and brown children wearing only a skimpy shirt - or nothing. Western or Japanese mountain climbers in heavy boots were occasionally seen among the natives. On "Freak Street" Western hippies were allowed, for a time, to indulge in drugs without interference from the Nepalese government, and became a tourist sight. I explored the city and countryside on foot, or rode a rickshaw.

"We seem to have our own private rickshaw," said a New Zealand couple at my hotel with amusement. "A Nepalese driver is apparently devoting his services exclusively to us. Every morning we find him waiting outside the hotel gate. As we shop or walk around town, he follows patiently until we are ready to return to the hotel."

When the New Zealand couple left Nepal, to my surprise, I inherited their rickshaw driver, a friendly boy with a fun-loving sparkle in his big brown eyes. When I tried to walk he would pedal persistently along beside me, good-naturedly extolling how cheap it would be to ride. Sometimes I resisted, enjoying the walk, but I would eventually succumb to his persuasion and climb in his rickshaw. The driver called me Grandmother, under the impression this was a flattering term for a woman of my age. After a few days I began to understand his dogged devotion to one tourist at a time. He had once served as a Sherpa on a mountain climbing expedition. Someone in the group became fond of him, and flew him to California for a backpacking trip in the Sierras. It had been a fabulous adventure for a Nepalese boy, and I'm sure he hoped something equally wonderful might happen again.

I loved riding the rickshaw. When we went down hill, I clutched the sides with both hands. We careened wildly along, dodging chickens, dogs, goats, cows and naked children. The horn honked constantly, as both the driver and I laughed with delight. When we went uphill I felt sorry for him and got out and walked. In fact, on very steep hills I got behind and pushed. I probably presented an amusing picture in my flowered pantsuit and the beautiful cone-shaped hat, decorated with bright straw flowers, which I'd bought in Thailand. Actually, no one seemed to pay any attention as Grandmother pushed that rickshaw up the dusty, narrow, crooked streets of Katmandu. The driver would call happily over his shoulder,

"See Grandmother, this very bad road. Maybe you give me extra rupee this time?"

He saw no reason why Grandmother shouldn't help push the rickshaw, and even pay extra for the privilege. I gave him several extra rupees.

*   *   *

After several weeks in Nepal, the day arrived for my overland bus tour to depart. I met the people with whom I would spend the next three months on a circuitous route through Asia, Russia and Europe to England. Most were young Australians and New Zealanders. Six of us were of retirement age, and we wondered uneasily how we would fit in with that exuberant bunch of young people. However, no one seemed to pay any attention to age differences. Mirrors were scarce in second-class, Asian hotels, and we older travelers soon forgot we weren't the same age as our young traveling companions. When the young Aussies sang bawdy songs, we joined them, and we laughingly attempted the uninhibited contortions of dancing to rock'n roll in noisy Asian discotheques with flashing colored lights.

We drove down out of the Himalayas and through northern India, stopping every day to visit exquisite monuments and temples, including the Taj Mahal. We rode a boat on the Ganges at sunrise. Along the banks people bathed, washed clothes, stood on their heads practicing Yoga, chanted religious music and cremated their dead. As we walked the ancient, narrow streets of Varanasi, the Indian guide warned us to beware of cow-dung, pickpockets, aggressive peddlers, beggars and the ubiquitous scrawny cows. When we felt overwhelmed by the hoards of people, we retreated to the secluded, walled garden of our hotel, a building of decayed elegance left over from British occupation. The red velvet drapes had obviously been in the dining room for more than a century. Silent, white-clad Indians waited upon us, as mice scurried about the edges of the room. No one disturbed the lizards on the walls. They were said to eat the mosquitoes, which arrived in swarms after dark.

It was early spring and the Indian countryside was lush and green. A tattered goatherd, or a lone woman in a faded sari walking across a field with a clay jar on her head looked picturesque, but when we approached a village we encountered the ever-present, depressing, tightly packed throng of humanity which seems to be India. People converged from all directions to surround the bus and stare at us. Sometimes they laughed at the bus full of strange looking Westerners.

One whiff of Indian toilets, and we put away our modesty and used the fields as the Indians did, especially when we were suffering from "Delhi belly".

"Men to the right of the road, and ladies to the left," the tour guide would announce. One day a busload of Indians, several hundred yards away on an infrequently traveled road, spotted us, a dozen Western women squatting in a ditch. They honked and laughed and waved. It was difficult to know how to react in such an undignified position.

We drove back up into the Himalayas to Kashmir. Huge waterfalls cascaded down from the snow-covered peaks above. We encountered washouts, where great sides of mountains had given way, taking the road with it. The bottom of the gorge lay thousands of feet below. Wrecks of trucks and busses lay scattered down the slope. At the most dangerous stretches we got out and walked. The bus and driver laboriously made their way along the narrow road being bulldozed out of the mud and rocks. We reached the snow level, and finally a six-mile tunnel. Emerging upon a dazzling, snow covered slope, we looked down and saw the fruit trees in bloom, and the green valley and blue lakes of Kashmir.

During the British Raj, the English relished the cool climate of Kashmir for a holiday from the heat of India. The proud, independent Kashmirians refused to sell land to foreigners, so the British built big elaborate houseboats and floated them on the lakes. Kashmir now accommodated tourists in replicas of those houseboats, filled with intricately carved Victorian furniture and oriental carpets. Transportation around the valley was provided by *shikaras*, little canoes full of cushions and covered with a ruffled canopy. There were no motor driven craft on those high mountain lakes and streams, and the silence was crisp and lovely. I shared a houseboat with five of the young Australians while in Kashmir. Playfully affecting accents and mannerisms of nineteenth-century English Colonials, we "dressed" for dinner. Akbar, our dignified Kashmirian host, solemnly served us. At night we found hot water bottles in our beds. We didn't see much of the other members of the tour during our five days in Kashmir.

We boarded the bus to go back down out of the mountains. Bill, one of the older Australians, had become ill. Pale and breathing with difficulty, he sat on the bus in his usual silence. Before this three-month bus-trip was over we all became like intimate family members, but we didn't know Bill. His wife, Celia, was a non-stop talker. She spoke with a beautiful British accent, in a low voice, but she was like the relentless drone of a well-oiled motor. She had developed techniques that allowed no one to politely escape once she began one of her monologues. Bill and Celia always sat together on the bus. Bill looked out the window and nodded occasionally, while Celia talked.

Celia was silent now, worried about her husband. She called a doctor in the town where we stopped for the night and obtained an antibiotic. Bill improved somewhat. Lahore, Pakistan, was the next city with scheduled air flights, and Celia and Bill decided to leave the tour there and return to Australia.

As we were about to leave Lahore for the Khyber Pass, Bill died, unexpectedly, in his hotel room. We all stood by the bus in stunned silence on that hot, humid morning when we heard of Bill's death. Robyn, a young British tour-guide trainee, spending a few weeks with the tour, would stay behind to help Celia. The bus and tour would continue on schedule.

Another woman really should stay with the poor lady too, I realized. My own husband had died five years before, and even though Ike's illness had given some warning, I remembered those feelings of loss and vulnerability. For me, crossing the Khyber Pass was a highlight of the trip. I would have preferred going over with a camel train if I'd known how a lone woman of my age might arrange such a thing. Nevertheless, I was looking forward to the bus trip. If I stayed behind with Celia, I'd probably have to fly over the Khyber Pass to catch up with the tour. I waited, wishing someone else would offer, but no one did. I was the only single, older woman on the tour, and I finally volunteered. Staying behind was a nightmare at first, but the decision would eventually reward me with some of my most treasured memories.

Celia was in her hotel room. Bill's body lay by the bathroom door, where anyone entering had to step over him. Robyn went off to try to find out what we should do next. All I could do for Celia was listen.

"You are ever so generous to remain behind, Bertie. I'm exceedingly grateful. Bill used to say I'd talk to a lamppost if I couldn't find anyone to listen, and I must confess the truth of his observation. People assure me I don't speak with an Australian accent though. I had elocution lessons as a child, you see. How will I live without my darling? I thought he was better. Then this morning after "brekkie" he just collapsed on the floor. 'Don't leave me, Darling,' I said, 'Not here in this heathen land.' But he was gone—"

The door opened, and a hotel employee stuck in his head.

"Remember to keep the fan on," he warned. "Bodies deteriorate fast in this climate."

I didn't usually attend funerals and hadn't seen many corpses. I looked at Bill's body. Could it suddenly begin to deteriorate? Maybe I was getting more adventure than I'd bargained for.

"Can't someone pick him up off the floor," I asked. He returned with two Pakistanis who put Bill's body on one of the twin beds.

"I phoned my children in Australia," Celia continued. "'Bill passed away,' I told them. My daughter-in-law said, 'Oh no Mum!' She agreed I should continue on with the tour. There's no reason to return to Australia now. I'll get a refund on Bill's ticket, you know. After this horrible tragedy, loosing my dearest Bill, maybe I'll just treat myself to an emerald ring. I'll look for one in the Istanbul Bazaar. They say one can find wonderful bargains there. Bill wanted me to have this trip, you know. We've planned for years. All Englishmen should make at least one trip home during their lifetime, you see. I'm sure Bill would want me to continue on without him. 'Oh no Mum!' That's what my daughter-in-law said—"

Robyn returned and reported cremation was illegal in Pakistan, for religious reasons. Burial must take place the day of death, because of the climate. He had located an Anglican missionary who agreed to hold the funeral. We went to the police station to sign documents.

"Why must I sign anything? My poor darling just collapsed there on the *floor*. And in this strange land where one doesn't speak the language—"

The officials surrounding us didn't understand a word Celia was saying. They were shouting in Pakistani, convinced we would comprehend if they spoke loudly enough. Celia signed the papers and we returned to the hotel. Three tall, thin Pakistanis in dingy, white skirts, from which their long, thin, barefoot legs protruded, put Bill's body in a box covered with black plastic. They carried it out through the lobby and put it in an old Ford station wagon, crudely re-painted black. We rode to the cemetery with the missionary and his wife. Traffic on the streets of Lahore was crowded and hectic. Trucks, busses and motor scooters created a constant roar of noise. Camels, horses, oxen, water buffalo and donkeys pulled carts and wagons.

A high brick wall surrounded the Christian cemetery where the British had interred their loved ones. There, except for the murmur of distant traffic, it was quiet. The sound of birds, and the creaking wheels of the wooden cart, upon which the Pakistani men placed Bill's coffin, broke the silence. A few unkempt flowers grew under the huge old trees. The missionary wore a long white embroidered robe, which moved gently in the slight breeze. We stood by the open grave and read scriptures together. In the traffic on the way back to the hotel Celia talked to the missionary's wife.

"You are ever so courageous to live out here and work among the heathen."

"One does what one must when one does the Lord's work, doesn't one—"

"I'm thankful to leave my dear husband in a Christian cemetery. If one can manage, one should always leave one's loved ones among one's own kind, *shouldn't* one, even in uncivilized parts of the world. You have been most comforting, really, most comforting. It was a lovely funeral though, wasn't it—?"

"It was quite lovely," injected the missionary's wife. The missionary nodded solemnly. Those quiet moments in the cemetery had been a peaceful respite in that nightmare of a day.

Back at the hotel the nightmare resumed. The desk clerk expected me to share Celia's room and sleep in the dead man's bed. At my frantic insistence he finally gave us another room, one for three. It was to be shared by Celia, *Robyn* and me. Someone else would sleep in Bill's bed that night. I hoped the sheets got changed.

The tour we were on was incredibly cheap. The whole trip, including accommodations, had cost only a few hundred dollars. We slept four and five to a room. When the beds didn't come out even, a boy sometimes *bunked* in with some of the girls. The young Australians seemed to pay no attention to each other as they awoke in the morning and brushed their teeth in their knickers and nightclothes. So far the two older couples on the tour had been given their own rooms. So while I had accustomed myself to sharing, Celia was shocked to realize she was to sleep in the same room with Robyn.

"Really! What would my darling Bill think? His first night in the ground and I'm to sleep in the same hotel room with a man. Well! My poor dear must be positively turning in his grave. You don't suppose Robin will try to rape us, do you Bertie?"

He didn't. Unfortunately. That might have turned off Celia's motor. We went out to dinner and Celia told the waiter,

"My dear husband died today. Just fell by the bathroom door. I had to leave him here in Pakistan among the heathen, you know. We had a lovely funeral though—"

"Yes Ma'am," said the waiter.

Moslem men must have found Western women like creatures from another planet, with their bare arms and faces, and their bold and fearless manner, acting powerful enough to be men, rather than properly demure Moslem women. Hotel employees didn't appear surprised by anything Western tourists did or said.

Celia repeated her story to the waiter at "brekkie" the next morning, to the taxi driver on the way to the airport, and to everyone in the airport who understood English. Because of recent political unrest we were thoroughly searched. The discovery of a blond wig, false eyelashes and women's clothing in the suitcase Robyn was claiming caused some consternation.

"It's my dear, departed husband's suitcase," explained Celia indignantly. "Bill wanted me to be my usual glamorous self, even on the tour, and men don't need a whole suitcase, do they. I had to bury him here in Pakistan, you know, among the heathen—"

"Go get on the plane," the airport officials said hastily, probably not wanting to hear Celia's story again.

We had been unable to fly over the Khyber Pass, thank heavens, and were headed for Peshawar, a small town at the foot of the mountains. Robyn and I sat together, silently, resting our ears. Celia sat next to a beautifully dressed Pakistani woman. On landing in Peshawar, Celia introduced us to her seat companion. The woman was going to her niece's wedding. She felt sorry for Celia and invited us all to the *mendi*, a Moslem wedding feast held the evening before the wedding. Celia felt the party might lift her spirits. Robyn and I were thrilled by such a fabulous invitation, one that Celia had obtained for us by her incessant talking.

That evening we squeezed into an open, three-wheeled taxi and rode out into the suburbs to a Pakistani general's home. Thousands of Christmas tree lights lit the garden. A huge canopy had been erected and carpets placed on the ground. Musicians were playing strange, eerie-sounding, oriental instruments. Robyn was hurried into the house to join the men. A *mendi* was a women's party, and men and women did not mingle socially in Pakistan. The guests wore bright colored tunics embroidered with gold, silk trousers and long scarves. All displayed diamonds, rubies and emeralds, and the family fortune on their arms in the form of gold bracelets. The younger women took turns dancing, moving sensuously to the exotic Asian music. Other guests placed money on the dancers' heads, which fell to the carpets and was collected for charity. The bride was led out of the house for a few minutes. She was heavily veiled and sat hunched over, staring at the ground.

"What's wrong with her?" I couldn't help exclaiming.

"She's just shy," someone said, and they all laughed.

She looked about sixteen and terrified. An older, married sister of the bride was a medical student. Five of her classmates were at the party, all lovely, girls with smooth complexions, dark hair and eyes, and fine features. They spoke beautiful English and were eager to explain Pakistani customs. Marriages were arranged. The prospective bride was presented to the groom. He could reject her, but the bride only felt grateful not to be spurned. One Pakistani woman insisted such marriages were more successful than Western romantic matches were. Several of the medical students, who had their husbands chosen in this manner, agreed. One was not married, and declared her determination to select her own husband. The evening felt like an experience out of the Arabian Nights.

Robyn also enjoyed his time with the Pakistani men. Back at the hotel, he and I exchanged stories of the party over a cup of tea. We began talking to the friendly young recently wed waiter, who asked if Robyn was married.

Robyn said no, and the waiter asked sympathetically,

"Your family is doing nothing to find you a wife?"

"In my country we find our own wives," said Robyn.

"How much do they cost?"

"I suppose a marriage license costs about three pounds."

"Three pounds!" the waiter exclaimed. "If that were all they cost here, I'd surely have a dozen."

The waiter explained that in Afghanistan, the country over the Khyber Pass, wives were very expensive. Indeed, many Afghans lived their entire lives without affording even one. (A shortage probably caused by greedy rich men acquiring a dozen.)

The next day Robyn was able to buy the last three places on a color-fully painted, third class Afghan bus. We squeezed into the rear seat with three Afghan tribesmen. Baggage was piled on top of the bus. A box fell off from time to time as we bounced up the pass. The Afghan riding on top would pound on the roof, and the bus would stop. Someone would run back to retrieve the fallen luggage. Many Afghans were tall, handsome and fierce looking. Once, two tribesmen got into what seemed to be an acrimonious disagreement. The men all took off their belts. They were apparently ready to sling them like whips, using the heavy, metal buckles as weapons. To our relief the argument was settled without violence, and the men put on their belts again. (Russia and the United States were soon to give the Afghans machine-guns and rockets.)

Several times the bus stopped by a stream. The men jumped off and ran down to wash their feet and knelt on the rocks to pray toward Mecca.

The Khyber Pass was barren and rocky. I watched the nomads and camel-trains from the bus window. I might not be riding a camel, but I was crossing the Khyber Pass with a bunch of Afghan tribesmen. So much history had passed this way, traveling between Europe and the East. I suspected many things had not changed during the centuries. At the summit we stopped, and everyone paid a fee to the local tribesmen "to ensure our safety across the pass". One of the men near us on the bus spoke a little English.

"Where you from?" he asked.

"America," I answered, smiling at him.

"Ah, America!" he exclaimed, as he grabbed my hand and shook it. "How many husbands you got?"

"Two." I certainly wasn't going to admit I didn't have one, and maybe two would be even more of a put off.

"Good! I meet you tonight, your hotel," he announced. "Ten o'clock."

I must confess I felt touched to have a handsome young tribesman try to make a date with me at my age. Nevertheless I stayed close to an amused Robyn until we reached Kabul, and didn't smile at any more Afghan tribesmen. Afghan women wore a tent-like garment in public. They peeked out through a gauze-covered hole, to ensure that no man but their husband would get a glimpse of even their eyes. I wasn't sure Afghans could distinguish between a sixteen-year-old and a sixty-year-old woman. I sensed the power women of a traditional culture possess, exerting a potent effect upon sex-starved men by doing nothing more than being women. Some might have been reluctant to exchange such heady power for mere liberation. And who knows? If Western men had succeeded in their professed intention to "protect and take care" of women, perhaps we would have also been content to remain "little girls".

We caught up with our tour in Kabul. They were eating in a restaurant, the Istanbul Cafe. A delicious meal, including homemade

American pie, cost about seventy-two cents. The restaurant was dim and smoky, and packed with tourists. Asian music blared from a radio, and faded posters covered the walls. Celia sat at the end of the long table, next to some other Westerners. One of them asked if she was enjoying her trip.

"It's marvelously fascinating. We attended a Pakistani *mendi* last night. My traveling companions are most considerate. You see, my husband died day *before* yesterday and—"

The waiter arrived, and the tourists sat speechless, with dazed expressions on their faces, as Celia turned to give her order.

Then she continued, "I miss him terribly. But there's no reason to return to Australia. One keeps busy and has less time to think, doesn't one."

Celia did have time to think, though. I'd heard her crying at night when she was alone. She was struggling to continue her life without her husband. Whatever her failings, she had the courage of an elderly Australian woman determined to reach her mother country.

In Kabul we were told all tourists must be out of Afghanistan before the end of the month, as a revolution was scheduled to take place. We were in Iran, exploring the ruins at Persepolis, the ancient Persian capitol, when the Russians entered Kabul—using weapons more deadly than belt buckles.

The tour continued through Iran and Turkey, and our group became even more cohesive. The tour guide was a charming, educated, handsome Scotsman called Haggis. During the bus rides he lectured about the languages, history and customs of the areas through which we drove. The tour company appreciated their brilliant tour guide, but didn't entrust him with expense money for the entire trip. He collected funds sent from England to a local bank on the first of each month. Haggis knew a lit'l wee pub in every town in Asia. In fact, it was probably because of his fondness for lit'l wee pubs that the tour ran out of money near the end of each month. We would leave Haggis behind at some hotel until the tour company sent money to pay the bill. The bus and driver continued on to our next destination. By traveling all night, Haggis caught up with us.

One evening in eastern Turkey Haggis organized a costume party at a discotheque, in the basement of a former monastery. I dressed as an Easter Bunny, in pink flannel pajamas, with a wad of toilet paper for a tail and a pink scarf for ears. At 2:00 AM, I found myself dancing with an amorous Turkish carpet merchant. He seemed to be nursing a fantasy that some Western woman would find his charms irresistible and carry him off to the legendary pleasures of the affluent West. In earnest imitation of a five-feet four-inch Omar Sharif, he tried to convince each of us he had fallen suddenly and madly in love.

Could anyone possibly claim my life had been unhappy, I reflected blissfully. On the contrary, I had surely led a charmed life. How else could I have been so lucky to have stumbled upon this unique tour and have such fun at my age?

After Greece we entered the Communist-block countries at Bulgaria, then Rumania and finally Russia. One couple, on another tour traveling with us, had been born in Russia and escaped. They left their tour before entering Russia, fearful the Communists might keep them if given the chance. The Cold War was intense at that time, and the KGB was a sinister symbol of terror. Haggis warned us to obey all rules, for Western justice would be unable to help us if we got into trouble. If we bought black-market rubles, he urged us to use them for something consumable, such as champagne and caviar. The border guards would search our luggage when we left Russia, to ensure that we didn't have more than could have been purchased with our officially exchanged rubles. We learned to elude the surveillance of the official tour guide assigned to us in each city, by splitting into two groups and going in different directions. Fraternizing with the Russians was rarely possible though, for few of them spoke English. One evening we found ourselves at a nightclub. The musicians, although unable to speak English, sang popular songs without accent and cowboy songs with an authentic Texas drawl. The music was slow and the dancing sedate.

"You should teach these Russians how to dance," I urged the young Australians, having myself recently learned the uninhibited wiggle young people called dancing.

The evening wore on, and the Russians drank vodka. The music turned frenzied. People began leaping and spinning, and squatting on one leg. A fight erupted. The police arrived and sent everyone home. The Russians all left docilely enough, but contrary to what we would have expected, they didn't appear to be afraid of the police.

We exited from Russia into Finland. As we traveled through Scandinavia, we stayed in youth hostels. In Copenhagen we stopped at an inexpensive hotel in the porno district. Continuing on toward Berlin, we left Haggis at the porno-district hotel waiting for money to pay the bill. As we arrived in Berlin we noticed the run down buildings, and feared we were lost, and had wandered into East Berlin. I was the only one who spoke any German and I kept jumping off the bus to ask the way to West Berlin.

"Straight ahead," was the answer.

Skeptical, and feeling a little apprehensive, we spotted two police on motorcycles and asked them to show us the way to West Berlin. They obligingly turned on their red lights, and escorted us right up to the east side of the Berlin Wall. The East German border guards were indignant and *angry*. How could they allow us into West Berlin when we had no papers showing that we had properly entered East Berlin? Phone calls brought East German officials in big black limousines, and they held a conference. We waited uneasily, wondering what they might do to us.

"It's not our fault," Celia said. "Your police were the ones who brought us here. Really! One would think they should know what they were doing. After all that has already happened to us on this trip. My poor Bill passing on and everything—"

Finally the two policemen got back on their motorcycles and took us to Checkpoint Charlie.

"Where on earth did you come from?" asked the American border guards. Check Point Charlie was a place through which East Germans tried to escape, and tour busses didn't appear there.

"India," drawled our Aussie bus driver laconically.

When we arrived in England, it was still Spring. We all stayed together in the same hotel for a week, reluctant to break up the close family we had become. At hotels during that three-month bus trip we occasionally encountered people on similar inexpensive bus tours. They invariably expressed envy at how much fun our group seemed to be having. Where were the irritations, rivalries, jealousy, vexations and personality clashes that usually afflict strangers thrown into such close contact? Why was there no sign of a generation gap? Why did we retirees feel at such ease with the young people? Lack of such strife would seem to contradict my belief that conflict plays a necessary and normal role in human experience. I haven't told the whole story. We had our conflict. No battle took place, but we actually had our own Cold War, "us" against "them". The tour company had originally planned two tours: one, the standard, inexpensive tour accommodating mostly young people. The other, called an Armchair Adventure, was for more mature and affluent travelers, and offered first class accommodations and restaurants. Each tour was under-subscribed, so the company decided to run both tours on the same bus, with one tour guide and one driver. When we arrived in a town, the bus would drive to a first class hotel, and we would wait while the Armchair Adventurers (soon renamed the "Arm-pits" by the young people) and their luggage were unloaded. Then we continued on to the center of the city for our more native accommodations. The two groups saw each other only on the bus, where they mixed about as well as oil and water. Some of the first class group were shocked by the tour guide's escapades in lit'l wee pubs with the young people, and they wanted classical music played on the bus stereo. The young people retaliated by singing bawdy songs. Even Celia, who would have actually felt more comfortable among the Armchair Adventurers claimed to share the young people's taste in music. Nothing promotes cohesiveness like a Cold War. There were some complainers among the first class travelers, and I'm sure there were also some very nice people. However, no one doubted our group was experiencing more of the countries through which we traveled. And maybe we felt obligated to have more fun.

I cherish that glimpse, no matter how brief and superficial, of other cultures. Only during this century of mechanistic materialism has it become fashionable to believe culture, like the soul, has no biological component. Culture has sometimes been thought of as a collection of ideas and attitudes acquired after birth, and not an integral part of people. Yet we have tried often enough to impose our Western culture on other people and failed, sometimes destroying them in the process.

I'm convinced much of my character, personality differences and attitudes were always with me, inherited from my ancestors. And whatever insight and maturity I personally have achieved was through the painful process of meeting challenges I wouldn't have chosen. If I had been given a choice.

CHAPTER 20

Should we wish that children never know unhappiness?

Guy to Siberia. (By our country, not the Russians.) After he became a physicist, the *National Academy of Science* sent him to the university at Novosibirsk for six months on a scientist exchange program. He fell in love with a Russian woman with two daughters. The Soviets kicked him out of the country. He managed to return and get married, and was again expelled. Returning to Novosibirsk once more, his wife became pregnant. He offered to live in Siberia with his family. The Soviets refused, probably feeling they were having enough trouble with their own dissident physicists. An American scientist would be a sure troublemaker. He was again ordered to leave the country. (He could have stayed in Russia if he had been willing to denounce the United States.)

The FBI learned of Guy's willingness to live in Russia and interviewed him. Guy told them nationalism was the biggest cause of the world's problems, and since he had no materialistic ambitions, and wouldn't be bothered by the austere Soviet living standard, the world would benefit from an American scientist living in the Soviet Union.

"Where did you get such a weird attitude?" asked the shocked FBI agent. "From your parents?" Russia was still our mortal enemy, and willingness to live there was considered treason.

Not sure he could convince the FBI agent he thought up his own weird ideas, Guy ventured,

"From my father, I guess." It seemed a safe answer, since Ike could no longer be censured for any of his son's unorthodox attitudes.

The FBI agent kept Guy under surveillance, interviewing him several times during the next year. Finally, the Soviets allowed Guy to bring his family to the United States. After three years and so many trips on *Aeroflot*, he was penniless when they finally arrived in California. I had just returned from a year in the South Pacific and was living in a small apartment. I hurriedly found a place large enough for all of us. After living with me for six months, and working as a short-order cook, Guy obtained a position at a college and moved his family to Pennsylvania. He quickly acquired materialistic ambition; mere survival began to challenge him. His wife is a beautiful girl, sweet and affectionate, and seemed happy to cope with an absent-minded physicist, but Russians don't understand money. In Russia, consumer goods, such as a roll of toilet paper or a bottle of perfume, had value; money had very little. Russians didn't get evicted for not paying the rent, and they didn't lose their job if they only showed up for work several days a week. As children they were taught that saving money was an evil, capitalistic pursuit. I watched in alarm as my Russian daughter-in-law when entering an American store, would exclaim excitedly,

"Oh, its every Russian woman's dream to find herself in a store like this!"

Guy was kept busy trying to provide for his increasing family of beautiful, Russian-speaking females. (They have two more daughters.) After Guy and his family left, I found myself alone in a three-bedroom apartment. I wondered if Tony might like to live with me again. He could attend the day-center for retarded people, which I'd noticed down the street. He had been free from emotional disturbances for several years, supposedly because of medication. (He was taking Valium, Lithium, Haldol - and finally, Artane to counter the side effects of all the antipsychotic drugs.) Excited at the thought of having him with me again, I made arrangements for Tony, aged thirty, to move from the board-and-care home.

Children labeled autistic generally grow up with some degree of retardation, and I can only speculate what those psychologists who first examined Tony had in mind when they insisted he was "extremely bright". Perhaps they suspected a condition now known as Asperger's Syndrome, a term applied to adults with average or above average intelligence and unusual personalities. The similarities of people labeled Asperger's Syndrome and those called autistic are in how they relate (or don't relate) to people. Maybe psychologists once believed autistic children grew up to be adults with Asperger's Syndrome, and that psychotherapy could ensure that all children would grow up with average personalities.

Temple Grandin, an animal psychologist at the University of Colorado, has been called Asperger's Syndrome. I've read much that she has written, and seen her on TV. Sometimes she describes her "differences", and I realize my reaction would be similar to hers - not the way an "average" person would react. Yet, I consider my reaction merely my own individuality, and she considers hers evidence of "dysfunction". For instance, "small talk". I can force myself to participate, clumsily, but talking merely to be sociable is a chore for me. (Now that I am approaching eighty, I can turn off my hearing aid and claim I don't hear.) Other members of my family are even worse. My brother becomes visibly distressed at having to sit through more than fifteen minutes of pointless social conversation. Tony is capable of saying anything he wishes, but he avoids conversation whenever possible. One of my hobbies is Tournament Bridge. Unusual personalities are common among serious bridge players, and some might well be regarded as "Asperger's". Playing bridge is a way to relate to people without conversation.

Adolescence is the time when all of us try to come to terms with our individuality, and I suspect some pain is involved for most of us. I even think the pain is a healthy part of the process. My own "shyness" and inability to understand other people's thinking lasted into adulthood, and wasn't really resolved until my traumatic encounter with the psychologists. Perhaps some adolescents find it easier to attribute their problems to Asperger's Syndrome, rather than normal human variability. Personally, I would resist if anyone tried to label me some syndrome, insisting I am as "normal" as people born with average personalities.

When Tony returned to live with me as an adult, I had stopped trying to change him and accepted him as he was. The expression on his face was not as bright and alert as when he was a child, and people now usually realized he was retarded. I've heard anti-psychotic medications damage the brain, but maybe, like most adults, Tony merely lost the natural curiosity and playfulness of childhood. He was easier to live with, but I couldn't help thinking wistfully of the imaginative little imp he used to be.

Tony's biggest difference from other retarded people is his lack of complicated emotions. He experiences anger and fear, but seems to lack feelings such as jealousy, pride, embarrassment, ambition, envy, shame and feelings of inferiority. He feels no urge to achieve, no desire to be like other people. He is glad to see his brother and sister, but appears unconcerned if he doesn't see them for months or even years at a time. When Ike died Tony became aware we were grieving and asked,

"What happened to poor old Daddy?"

We explained Daddy died. Once, when questioned about one of his fears, Tony replied that he didn't want to die, so he apparently had some understanding of death. However, Tony never again asked about his father. He is always glad to see me, and when I die he will miss the things I do for him, but I doubt he will grieve. I suppose I should really feel glad about that.

"What'll happen if Tony cries like a baby?" he sometimes asked.

"People might not like you," was the only answer I could come up with.

Tony would laugh. Maybe he thought this was funny because he wasn't sure what "not liking someone," meant.

Tony did sometimes cry like a baby. He cried when I disciplined him by denying him a candy bar, or over something he feared, such as riding a bus or boat. When he saw a dog, he cried and clung to me for protection, looking pretty silly since he towered over me and outweighed me by eighty pounds. Most people are not afraid of little boys, but strange acting men frighten everyone. I worry someone who fears Tony might harm him, and he is defenseless. Tony has always been treated with kindness, and people are one thing he does not fear.

Unlike most retarded men, Tony has strong sex drives and masturbated since puberty. Imposing enough inhibitions that he did it in private was difficult. Once, when he was about nineteen, he was home from the state hospital for the weekend. We went to the newsstand for a copy of *Disneyland* magazine. Tony still enjoyed stories about Snow White, Cinderella and Peter Pan. On this particular day the newsstand was out of *Disneyland*, and I suggested *Woody Woodpecker* instead.

"No," said Tony, "I want a book about naked ladies."

"Oh Tony, don't you like Woody Woodpecker any more?" I asked.

Tony repeated his demand for naked ladies in a voice that could be heard all over the store. A nearby customer, apparently amused by a grown man's preference for *Playboy* instead of *Woody Woodpecker*, suppressed a smirk behind the magazine he was examining. I left the store in embarrassment. Tony followed, still demanding naked ladies.

On the whole, I enjoyed the responsibility of caring for Tony during the year he lived with me. He woke me at four o'clock on Easter morning.

"The Easter bunny came, Mom. The Easter Bunny came!" (I once told Tony there was no Santa Claus, deciding he was too old for such things. He didn't believe me.)

Then one day at the day center, for no apparent reason, Tony knocked down other handicapped people and tore up his clothes. I doubt these violent episodes had any cause, other than something within Tony. He has had them every few years throughout his life. We increased his medication, but it was obvious all those antipsychotic drugs he was taking were not what had been preventing his "disturbed" behavior. Tony was expelled from his day program, and his social worker was unable to find another. He stayed home with nothing to do but look at television. One evening while I was out, Tony kicked holes in the walls, broke mirrors, chairs, lamps, and smashed all the dishes. This time his "disturbed" behavior was apparently deliberate, for he laughed at my distress upon seeing my demolished apartment. I had to place him in a psychiatric hospital. My sense of failure was again painful, and I shed more tears.

When I explained Tony had apparently smashed a bathroom mirror with his fist, the hospital admissions officer said,

"Tony! Don't you know that's dangerous?"

"Oh I was careful," Tony assured him. "Tony was careful, Mommy." He didn't want anyone to think he'd do something dangerous.

Tony was again admitted to a state hospital for a year, after which he was put on a new assortment of antipsychotic drugs and assigned to another group home. He has continued taking drugs, and is now obviously addicted to them.

Tony, now forty, lives in a board-and-care home in a nearby town. (I had re-applied, and Tony was accepted by the Regional Center.) Such homes, operated by individuals and caring for up to six retarded people, have replaced institutions. They can be good, bad or mediocre, depending upon the person who runs them. Regional Center supervision tries to eliminate the worst. However the really bad ones, interested in maximizing profit, can even skimp on food. Fortunately, the home in which Tony now lives, happens to be one of the best.

*   *   *

Twentieth-century psychiatrists and psychologists are not the only ones who seem to regard people alteration as one of their skills. Despite lack of evidence for the effectiveness of such efforts, many people in our society devote their lives to trying to change other people. Personally, I've found my ability to change anyone, including my children, to be minuscule. However, most of us have some ability to deliberately change ourselves. (At least those of us who believe in free will do.) In fact, the changes we make in ourselves might be the qualities of which we should feel proud, instead of those talents bestowed upon us by nature. When my daughter moved from the house where she lived for the first five years of her marriage, she admitted a nostalgic affection for the place where she had accomplished so much. Her son was born while she lived there. She achieved a relationship with her stepson. Becoming a successful nurse, she acquired enough assertiveness to work as a supervisor. She decided she had inherited the family tendency toward alcoholism, and joined a support group for recovering alcoholics. (Surely a successful "recovering alcoholic" is a stronger person than someone who never had to confront the problem.) It was in this house Sherry finally managed to quit smoking, resorting to hypnotism, acupuncture, support groups and any other help suggested. Then, gaining twenty pounds, she had to learn to diet. Both Guy and Sherry suffer from occasional mild depression. Sherry once tried psychiatry, but decided looking for "reasons" further depressed her. She has found that exercise, abstinence from alcohol, and acceptance of the condition helps her cope with her increasingly rare down-cycles. Although an advocate of support groups, I think she is proud of her achievements. She is a busy woman, involved with her family, her career, holistic medicine, friends and a business she is starting. Indian shamans are among her friends, and she spends many of her vacations participating in Native American ceremonial dances. She is tolerant; open disagreement with anyone would be contrary to her nature. Nevertheless Sherry decides the significance of ideas for herself, and is often as unorthodox as her mother.

If it were in my power, I would have presented all my children with safe, pleasant lives, free from pain and suffering. I would probably have spared them their most stressful challenges—if it had been within my power. I was able to do that only for Tony. The other two have encountered problems and had to struggle, sometimes quite a lot. They have both grown into mature, responsible adults. Both Guy and Sherry feel a need to do something with their lives that might make the world a little better, a need stronger than their desire for material possessions. Their view on questions of right and wrong sometimes differs from mine, and they are sometimes more altruistic and unselfish than I.

I don't believe I taught my children to be moral; it was an intrinsic part of their natures, the accumulated result of all the effort, pain and growth experienced by their ancestors.

CHAPTER 21

Did Freud, Marx and Darwin represent 20th century materialism?

Today, some psychiatrists might still encourage normal, but unhappy adults to remember a traumatic childhood, but few still believe mother causes her child's mental illness. The influence of Freud had upon American thinking is difficult to explain. Maybe novelists were responsible. Psychiatric formulas made handy plots.

Bruno Bettelheim, proponent of "maternal rejection" as the cause of autism, committed suicide in 1990. He was a self-proclaimed psychologist and psychoanalyst. He came to this country during the Second World War when scholastic credentials from Europe couldn't be verified, and invented a long list of academic achievements. Becoming a world-famous writer and professor at the University of Chicago, Bettelheim directed the Sonia Shankman Orthogenic School for disturbed children. A survivor of the Holocaust, he reached his conclusion about the cause of autism by describing how inmates of concentration camps sometimes exhibited autistic behavior. Bettelheim suggested mothers might affect their autistic children like Nazi prison guards. After the war he searched for emotionally superior children raised on kibbutzim in Israel. He hoped to find children uncontaminated by mothers. After Bettelheim's death, his fraudulent academic credentials were revealed. Some of his "cured" patients declared they were never mentally ill in the first place. Other former patients accused Bettelheim himself of physically and verbally abusing them. As for the eighty-five percent success rate he claimed, Bettelheim didn't conduct follow-up studies. Whenever Bettelheim needed a statistic in order to obtain funding, he merely made one up.

I never managed to track down any specific research in which Tony might have been involved. I once wrote the Army and asked if Tony had been a part of any research project. They replied they had examined the records of the Child Guidance Clinic for the years between 1961 and 1963, but our names were not in the records. It was obvious those army psychologists wished they had never heard of us, but I hadn't realized they could delete us from their medical records. The Army referred me to the Surgeon General. Someone from that office suggested that, if my son had been involved in research, the records were probably destroyed when the project was completed.

A friend in Marin County was acquainted with the woman, long since retired, who had been director of the nursery school to which Tony was denied admission when he was seven years old. My friend arranged meeting for me. The social worker who also interviewed us at the March-of-Dimes clinic had been the woman who accused me of allowing Tony to vegetate, and stated he must be under the care of a psychiatrist to attend the school. I had never met this woman who had been the director of the school at that time.

"I'm no longer bitter because Tony was denied admission," I assured her. "It's just that I could more easily accept the things which happened to us if I knew for certain they were caused by research." The incident had occurred twenty-five years ago, before the passage of a law requiring parents' informed consent for involving children in research. I hoped this woman might now be candid.

She didn't remember Tony. "All parents of handicapped children need psychiatric counseling," she declared defensively. She assured me the nursery school had not received funding from any government agency, Federal or local. Not one penny! However she did concede that most of the children had received scholarships. She mentioned the names of the two psychiatrists who had read my manuscript. The doctor who diagnosed Tony as schizophrenic for the Regional Center and then refused to discuss his diagnosis, and the psychiatrist who charged me half-price for the advice to "tell Dr. Dingle exactly what I thought of him" had both been on the board of directors of the school. Nonetheless, no one concerned with the school had been involved in research of any kind. Absolutely not!

I've since of many destructive experiments psychiatrists have performed, and are still performing. Actually, any drug or surgical procedure prescribed by a psychiatrist is experimental; there is no known cure for mental illness. There is not even a scientific definition of the term. Many "mentally ill" patients recover, with or without treatment. Few if any scientific follow up studies are conducted to see whether psychiatric "treatments" harm or help. Only after thousands of lobotomies did the public finally notice doctors were turning people into zombies.

An experience I had on a ship in the South Seas convinced me of the futility of claiming I'd been the victim of a research conspiracy. I met a woman, an English lady of about my age, in the ship's library. I was examining a book on the Middle East. She mentioned she had a son in Saudi Arabia, a physicist.

"What a coincidence," I said. " I have a son in Siberia. He's a physicist."

We formed one of those instant friendships lone travelers sometimes achieve. We discussed politics, religion and the educational systems of the countries with which we were familiar. She told about her child-hood in China, where her parents were missionaries. They had escaped to Singapore at the beginning of World War II, and from there managed to get to Australia. When I met her on the ship, she was returning to England, where she'd been born.

"My husband died recently, and I feel lost without him," she explained a few days after we met. We were having a drink in the lounge after a day ashore in Bali.

"My husband died ten years ago, and I miss still miss him," I agreed.

"There are other reasons I had to get away from Australia," she said.

I sipped my drink and waited with interest for her to explain.

"Well, you see I had some bad experiences with doctors."

"I can relate to that. I've had my troubles with the medical profession."

She glanced at me uneasily and then looked away. "Most people don't believe me when I describe what happened to me."

"Oh I'll believe you! People didn't believe me either," I said. "I felt helpless in my confrontations with doctors."

"Well, actually—the truth is— they were experimenting on my mind."

"Really!"

"They put listening devices in my home," she continued earnestly. "They even put an infrared camera in the ceiling over my bed."

I looked at her closely. She didn't seem to be joking. Pleasant and cheerful, there had been nothing to distinguish her in manner or appearance from other women our age. Until now.

"And finally, they began listening in on my thoughts," she continued. "I know because they were re-broadcasting them over BBC. Why I even heard my thoughts broadcast over radios of ships at sea!"

I'd promised to believe her, and tried to look sympathetic. She was the most interesting woman I'd met on the ship. I hope no psychiatrist ever got his hands on her and put her on some mind-altering drug.

Sometimes people behave irrationally and are a danger to themselves or others, and have to be restrained. While someone has to make that judgment, I'd have more faith in a panel of my peers than a psychiatrist. Psychiatrists and psychologists know no more about human motivation and thinking than the rest of us do, and they are continually looking for deviation from "normal". Psychiatry is the product of twentieth-century materialism. Life was thought to be without purpose, an accidental, mechanical process, reducible to simple formulas of cause and effect. Freud, Marx and Darwin replaced traditional religions. "Brain doctors" were the mechanics who fixed the mind. These mind-doctors also proposed treating the non-mentally ill—to make the machine run more efficiently. Free will has no place in a machine, and many materialists of this century suggest free will is an illusion, and doesn't really exist. Materialists are convinced that what most of us believe to be free choice is merely the inevitable result of molecules and neural connections in our brain. Socio-biologists even declared love and altruism to be "survival instincts" which became a part of our nature by "random mutation and natural selection".

Materialism is philosophy, not science. However, during the twentieth century many people accepted materialism as "scientific truth".

              *   *   *

Tony was forty-one, and I had moved to southern California. Sherry called one night and said Tony was in the hospital and not expected to live. He had been operated on for some kind of aneurysm in the bowel and stomach, but the damage was too extensive to repair. I drove all night to reach the Bay Area. It was as good a way as any to spend that awful night. Tony was still alive, but the doctors said he probably would not survive being taken off the respirator. When it was disconnected, we sat numbed with dread, listening to Tony's labored breathing. However, hour-by-hour his breathing slowly became stronger and more regular.

Finally Sherry said, "There is a cafeteria across the street if you get hungry."

Tony suddenly regained consciousness and tried to get out of bed.

"Tony, where are you going?" we exclaimed, for he was attached to a tangle of tubes and wires.

"To the cafeteria," Tony said. Eating had always been his favorite pastime, and now he didn't have a whole stomach or intestine. Although Tony had regained consciousness, the doctors told us he would soon succumb to massive organ failure.

For the next three weeks I remained in the hospital room with Tony, and sometimes he was alert and at other times seemed hardly conscious. The doctors explained that when his lower bowel re-inflated, the bacteria there would cause a massive infection. He developed a fistula, a drainage from his bowel, which smelled awful. The doctors said he was dying of gangrene. We signed a "no code", agreeing that they not try to resuscitate Tony if his heart stopped. Someone asked us to think about making arrangements for disposal of the body. People of normal understanding would have died of despair by this time. However Tony, who had no comprehension of what was happening to him, didn't succumb to any of these things. Sherry, a nurse, performed therapeutic touch, asked her friends to perform the procedure, asked Indian Shamans and friends all over the US and Mexico to pray for her brother. She insisted he be given antibiotics and nutritional IV. The doctors agreed, even though they regarded Tony's condition hopeless. After six weeks, Sherry had Tony transferred to UC Medical Center in San Francisco. Tony stayed there for the next seven months. He learned to get around the hospital with his IV pole, and one day he asked Sherry,

"Did MASH do this to me?"

She said yes, and the answer seemed to amuse him. We bought him the movie, and Sherry also got him a complete surgical outfit, including a mask and some goggles. He liked to dress up in it and go down and stand by the operating room door and greet the surgeons.

Once he stuck his head in the door and yelled, "Larry, are you in there?" Larry was the chief surgeon, and I doubt many of his patients called him by his first name.

I would never have thought Tony could tolerate all that happened to him and all that was done to him, but he adjusted to hospital life. Nearly everyone in the hospital knew him, and many of them seemed fond of him. He was a good patient, never complaining nor questioning any of the tests or procedures. The doctors were reluctant to operate on Tony a second time, perhaps because they were not optimistic of success. However the day finally came when he began to deteriorate from life on an IV, and a second operation was scheduled. The surgeons discovered that much of Tony's tissues had regenerated, and his recovery from a second operation was dramatic.

Since Tony's recovery, I've noticed him experience a delight and joy over things that I hadn't noticed before. Maybe he'd never before had anything bad to which he could compare his life. Perhaps he achieved something in recovering from his terrible illness, and like most personal growth, it wasn't achieved by being protected from "traumatic experiences".